BAID, HAKIM & DOCTORS
The Medicine Heritage of India

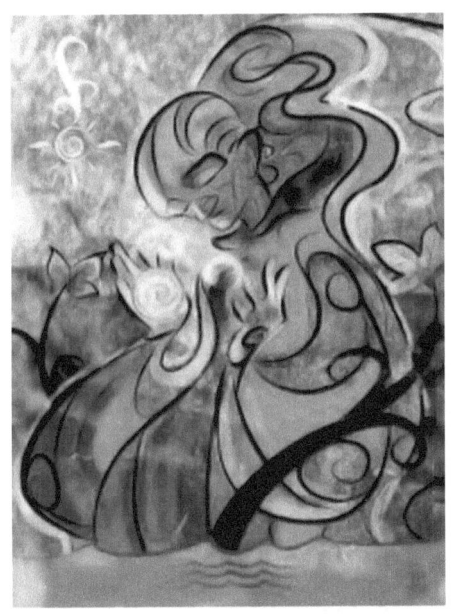

Dr Sanjay Sharma

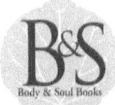

ISBN 978-93-81576-48-9
© Dr Sanjay Sharma, 2013
© Image: Jason Green, *The Healer* 2013

Editing   Abhijit Basu
Cover Design   Fravashi Aga
Layouts   Ajay Shah
Printing   Repro India Ltd

Published in India 2013 by
BODY & SOUL BOOKS
An imprint of LEADSTART PUBLISHING PVT LTD
Trade Centre, Level 1, Bandra Kurla Complex
Bandra (E), Mumbai 400 051, INDIA
T + 91 22 40700804   F +91 22 40700800
E info@leadstartcorp.com W www.leadstartcorp.com

US Office Axis Corp, 7845 E Oakbrook Circle, Madison,
WI 53717, USA

All rights reserved worldwide
No part of this publication may be reproduced, stored in or introduced into a retrieval system, or transmitted, in any form, or by any means (electronic, mechanical, photocopying, recording or otherwise), without the prior permission of the Publisher. Any person who commits an unauthorised act in relation to this publication can be liable to criminal prosecution and civil claims for damages.

Disclaimer The views expressed in this book are exclusively those of the Author and do not purport to be held by the Publisher.

ADVISORY
Please do not use any medication or method of treatment narrated in the book. Modern medicines are far more refined, safe and effective.

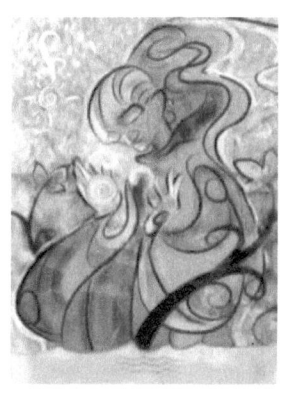

In loving memory of my daughter, Sakshi (23.09.94 ~ 11.12.12).

She always wanted to be a doctor...

and those she left behind ~ Samarth & Renu.

About the Author

DR SANJAY SHARMA is a consultant neurologist at Raipur Chhattisgarh, India. After completing his basic medical degree, he went on to do an MD in internal medicine. In 1994, he completed his training in neurology at PGI-Chandigarh.

Dr Sharma has written on the subjects covered in this book for various medical journals. When he is not working in his medical practice, he is deeply interested in research-based writing. Dr Sharma can be reached at: drsanjaysharma123@rediffmail.com

ADVISORY *Please do not use any medication or method of treatment narrated in this book. This is a work of historical research. Modern medicines are far more refined, safe and effective.*

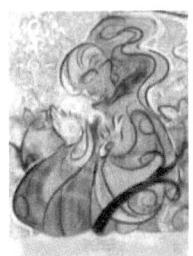

Contents

INTRODUCTION	7
1. MEDICINE	14
2. QUACKS, ILLNESS & SUPPORT	22
3. EPIDEMICS, INFECTION & PREVENTION	28
4. THE AUTUMN SCOURGE: MALARIA	34
5. DISAPPEARING DISEASES: SYPHILIS & YAWS	40
6. THE PERCEIVED CURSE: LEPROSY	45
7. LIVING IN HOPE: TUBERCULOSIS	51
8. WORMS IN THE GUT & BRAIN: NEUROCYSTICERCOSIS	54
9. FUNGUS	59
10. STIFF SPINE & TETANUS	62
11. HEAT, DUST & MENINGITIS	64
12. THE ANGRY GODDESS: SKIN SPOTS	69
13. DOGBITE & RABIES	72
14. SNAKEBITE	77
15. DEFORMITY	82
16. HYDROCELE TAPPING	87

17. THE NERVE-TRAPPING INJECTION 90
18. MEDICAL GEOLOGY: MANGANESE TOXICITY 94
19. SUN, MOON & WEATHER 97
20. DESPERATE SYMPTOMS CALL FOR
    DESPERATE REMEDIES: HEADACHE 103
21. EPILEPTICS IN LUNATIC ASYLUMS
    & DRUGS TO TREAT EPILEPSY 109
22. SEIZURES OF DIFFERENT KINDS 116
23. CHILDREN & GENES 122
24. THE DEFICIENT DIET 126
25. ADDICTION 131
26. SEX & LONGEVITY 140
IN CONCLUSION 144

Appendices 146
Glossary of Medical Terms 150
References 161
Photo Credits 173
Acknowledgements 174

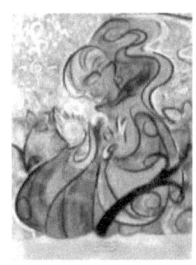

INTRODUCTION

FROM ITS GENESIS, THE SURVIVAL OF THE HUMAN RACE has been an epic saga of overcoming the myriad calamities of nature, thereby testing and tempering the resilience of this unique and intelligent life form. Kautilya's *Arthashastra*, dating way back to the 4th century BC, categorises calamities or acts of God, into eight broad types of sinister causality. The 'abominable eight' are: fire; flood; famine; disease and epidemics; rats; wild animals; snakes; and evil spirits. In ancient times, whenever a threat was encountered or perceived from any of these nefarious causalities, the King was expected to protect the people like a nurturing parent. However, more often than not, panic would set in, inducing the population to flee in a mass exodus, to escape the onslaught of the fearsome four – famine, fire, flood and disease.

Solutions to the other four problems – rats, wild animals, snakes, and evil spirits – included acquiring the skills to trap rats; developing weapons and poisons to fight wild animals; using herbal, native medicines to cure snakebite; and evolving complex rituals to ward off evil spirits. Significantly, faith and fear have led people to ascribe aspects of divinity to all four of these 'live' agents of human distress. Hence, rats, snakes, tigers, and any other deities or entities perceived to have a real or imagined potential to harm human beings, have been and continue to be, worshipped in temples and shrines all over India.

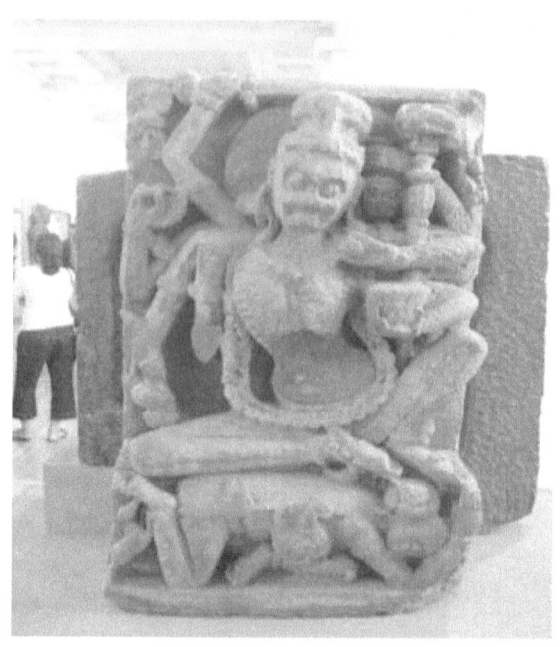

FIG 01: Statue of the Goddess Chamunda, Goddess of Destruction, Epidemics, Pestilent Diseases and Famine (courtesy: Wikipedia)

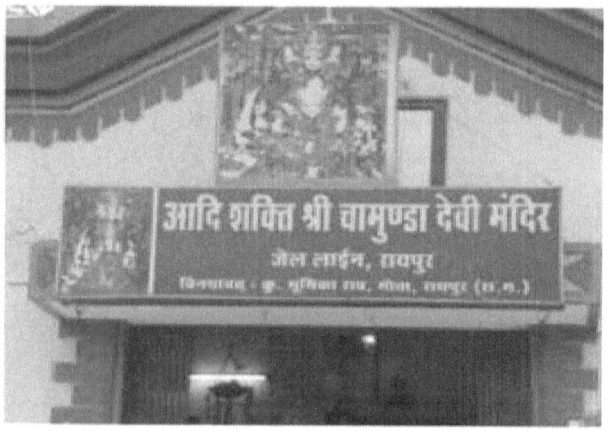

FIG 02: Temple of the Goddess Chamunda, located opposite the Medical College Hospital, Raipur, India

Indeed, a sense of sheer vulnerability led man to seek succour and protection from the deities, who often subsumed in their perceived divine forms, the very evil they are deemed to protect against. Thus, the Goddess *Chamunda* – with her emaciated frame, frightening face and bulging eyes – is associated with corpses and even sacrificial rituals. Her skeletal anatomy and jewellery made of bones, skulls and snakes, makes her image even more terrifying. These are the symbols of old age, death, decay and destruction. Her image is in marked contrast to the beauty of other goddesses conceived by Indian sculptors. But beauty in this case does indeed lie in the eye of the faithful beholder. *Devi Chamunda* – one of the seven Mother Goddesses (the *Saptamatrika*) – is invoked to protect against the many dangers that threaten Man on all sides, as can be seen in the imploring words of this talismanic verse: *evam dasha disho rakshet chaamunda shava-vaahanaa* (And let *Chamunda*, seated on a corpse, protect us on all ten sides) [1]. No wonder then, that the temple of the Mother Goddess in Raipur, located directly across from the Medical College Hospital, is widely accredited to hold out a divine assurance of salvation from disaster, for the populace.

There are several other striking illustrations of India's age-old quest for protection against disease and death through invocation of divine benefactors. Abiding faith in the Goddess *Sitala*, is said to provide immunity against smallpox and similarly, *Marhi Mata* protects her helpless, earthly devotees against the dreaded affliction of cholera. These are but two cases in point. In a more comprehensive sense, ancient Hindu society derived the necessary fighters' will and confidence to defeat and defy death by chanting the *Mahamrityunjaya mantra* (literally meaning 'Great Death-conquering hymn), which is dedicated to Lord *Rudra* (*Shiva*). The *mantra* ranks among the most famous Vedic hymns, and appears in the *Rigveda*, India's oldest and most sacred work, as also in the *Yajurveda*.

Ancient India's concern with disease and death did not, however, stop with the invoking of divine protection. Faith was supplemented by the efforts of pioneering practitioners of ancient *Ayurveda*, who themselves came to be revered as the worthy followers of *Dhanvantari* – the divine physician. In the course of such efforts, eminent *Ayurvedic* physicians like Nagarjuna and Vaag Bhatt, developed and perfected the science of Indian alchemy. The process involved purifying heavy metals converted into ash by soaking them in various liquids and heating them. Medicines made from these ashes and from plants, were used to cure various diseases. The ultimate goal of this old *Ayurveda*, was to make man immortal, a primordial urge in ancient civilizations. However, ethnic Indian research in this direction suffered a setback in the wake of Mohammedan invasions.

Yunani (Arabic) medicine, was introduced into India around 1350 AD. After the early Mohammedan conquests, there was a continuous influx of *Hakims* from Iran into India. Apart from their own medical science, they derived their knowledge partly from the Arabic translations of Greek authors. Great Sanskrit works were also translated into Arabic. The driving motivation behind such translations was the non-availability of the traditional Persian herbs in India, and the unsuitability of Greek medicines in the Indian climate[2]. *Yunani* medicines became the first choice although *Ayurveda* continued to survive with less importance. The practitioners of each school frequently borrowed from each other's prescriptions and secret recipes to treat the sexual asthenia of Royals and so impress them. However, after years of empirical treatment and sustenance of the profession through Royal patronage, they reached a plateau and failed to grow any further.

The East India Company's first fleet sailed towards the East in December 1600. It consisted of four ships, and each ship carried two surgeons. The Indian Medical Service (IMS) was formally constituted in January 1764. A number of Army medical officers arrived in India after a long intercontinental voyage from Europe and the United States. These scientists were fascinated by the new environment, its customs and diseases. They proposed many new theories on the causes of age-old diseases then prevalent in India.

After successive invasions of both armies and cultures from other lands, India became a melting pot of Asian and European medicinal metals, herbs and drugs. The traditional *Baid*, with his knowledge of *Ayurveda*; the *Hakim*, with his Persian healing touch; and the European doctors with newer inventions, competed with each other for supremacy[3]. 17th century European medicines were not superior to the *Yunani* and *Ayurvedic* formulations. In the pre-antibiotic era, there was hardly anything to choose between the Indian system and the European one. What the Europeans had, of course, was better surgical skill and the ability to treat the rampaging malarial fever with cinchona bark. Over the years, the British medical services displaced the indigenous science from its official status, as India saw the dawn of its own medical system, largely influenced by the British medical establishment – a system characterised by its network of dispensaries, hospitals, TB sanatoria and asylums.

After Independence, the traditional systems of medicine in India regained some of its lost ground. Today, India has multiple recognised systems of medicine. The *Yunani, Homoeopathy* and *Ayurvedic* systems are as much a part of Indian medical culture today as is the *Allopathic* system. And, as if to drive home the plurality of practices in Indian medicine, there are also large numbers of faith healers and quacks, serving the rural population. People have retained some faith in all forms of medicine and in their practitioners, ranging from quacks to doctors.

Diseases and healthcare services have changed very little in States like Chhattisgarh. In its geographical shape, the state resembles a seahorse without a tail. The tribal population resides in the northern and southern parts of the State. Chhattisgarh was part of the Central Provinces, under British rule. Raipur was one of the important towns of the Central Provinces,; it was not finally annexed to British India until 1854, when Nagpur State finally lapsed. Three years after Indian Independence in 1947, it became part of the State of Madhya Pradesh. The new state of Chhattisgarh was carved out of Madhya Pradesh, in November 2000 – a poor progeny of a weak mother State, because of its health status. The land of Chhattisgarh is rich in ores and minerals, with plenty of mining and industrial areas, and hence pollution-related diseases. Chhattisgarh, for all its natural riches, is inhabited by poor people, with roughly half the population living below the poverty line. In the tradition typical of India's demographically challenged states, Chhattisgarh's death and birth rates have always been amongst the highest in the country. The higher death rate, which earlier was partly attributable to frequent famines and epidemics, now reflects squarely on the poor health services available in the State.

I am one of ten neurologists who cover a population of over 20 million people. Like any other neurologist, my daily medical practice mostly revolves around out-patient (OPD) and the medical follow-up of patients with HAVES (Headache; Age-related arthritis of the spine; Vertigo (dizziness); Epilepsy; and Stroke). At our clinics, a group of chronic sufferers move from one person to another, offering herbal indigenous cures. Chronic headache is treated with *homeopathic* medication, and we consider it a safe treatment option, without rebound headaches or the side effects of painkillers. Neck and back pain is often managed by barbers and bone-settlers. Sufferers are treated by massage, manipulation or, at times, thumping/kicking the back. Malarial fever, illnesses of the gut, jaundice, joint pain and fractured bones, are all treated with herbs. Special oils are available to cure paralysis.

Every region uses particular words and methods to communicate and treat medical problems. For example, a lesion in the terminal spinal cord and roots was detected in a young tribal woman when she complained of an inability to sense her lover's touch on her buttocks. Such significant perceptions of patients' illnesses and the types of treatment offered to them since antiquity, constitute the central theme of this book (**Appendix-1**)

NOTES

1. *Markandeya-Puranam, Devi-kavacham,* verse 21

2. '*...At the same time, an opposition dispensary was opened under the charge of a Hakim from Cashmere, and for a time, the patients on their way to me were forcibly stopped and taken there for treatment; but as soon as this system was abandoned, the attendance at the Maharajah's Dispensary entirely ceased'.*
Cayley H. *Notes on Ladakh in 1867; Indian Medical Gazette;* January 1868, p. 3

3. '*Medicines locally available in the immediate surroundings will be suitable for people of that particular area. Even if a person resides in another place, the medicines of similar origin and properties should be used for him/her'.*
Astang Sangraha Sutra, pp. 23–35

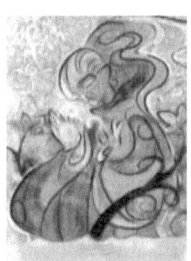
1 MEDICINE

In the 20th century, the ancient science of *Ayurveda* was falling behind in its bid to cope with the rapid advancement of European medical sciences. The period picture is reflected in the thoughts of the Father of the Nation, Mohandas Karamchand Gandhi, in his letter published in the *Indian Medical Gazette*, 1925:

My quarrel with the professors of the Ayurvedic system is that many of them, if not indeed a vast majority of them, are mere quacks pretending to know much more than they actually do, arrogating to themselves an infallibility and ability to cure all diseases . . . and in so doing, they have made it a stagnant system instead of a gloriously progressive science. I know of not a single discovery or invention of any importance on the part of Ayurvedic physicians as against a brilliant array of discoveries and inventions, which Western physicians and surgeons boast. In fact, Ayurvedic physicians' diagnoses as a rule consist in feeling the pulse, which I have known many to claim enables them to know even whether the patient is suffering from appendicitis. Whether the science of the pulse ever enabled ancient physicians to diagnose every known disease, no one can tell but it is certain that the claim cannot be sustained at the present moment. The only thing Ayurvedic physicians can safely claim is a knowledge of some vegetable and metallic drugs of great potency, which some of them succeed in administering for diseases they only guess and therefore often with much harm to their poor patients.

In India, *Ayurveda* was developed secretly, with religious overtones. But its structure and methods were evolved on secular and scientific lines, according to the best understanding of the scholar-practitioners of the day. *Ayurvedic* scholars classified most systemic diseases into four types. The basic three faults are related to the imbalance of five basic elements: *vaata* (air and ether), *pitta* (fire and water), and *kapha* (water and earth). Diagnosis of diseases was made based on descriptions of illnesses; and examinations consisted of the radial pulse being palpated at the base of the thumb, with three fingers. The character of the pulse was compared with the activities of the woodpecker to denote irregularities (*ectopics*), and the pace of birds like the quail or partridge denoted a faster rhythm. Despite the fact that they had little knowledge of the functioning of the brain, they adequately described epilepsy, headache and coma.

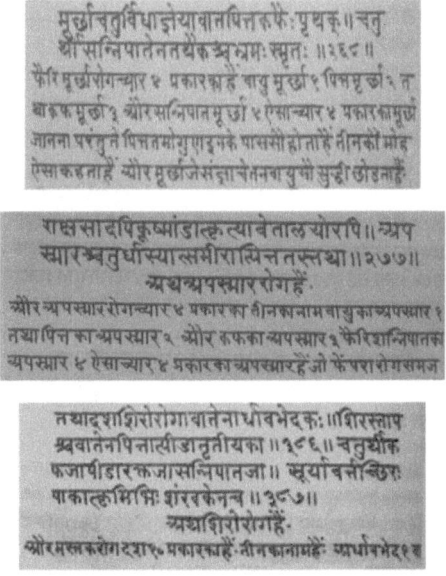

FIG 03: *Ayurvedic* text classified *Murchha* (loss of consciousness) and *Apasmara* (Epilepsy), as four types, due to a derangement of basic elements and 10 types of *Mastaka-roga* (headache), including one-sided headache (migraine).

Loss of consciousness was described as a cloudy appearance and a flow of colours in an empty space, before the patient fell to the ground like a wooden log. The colour (i.e. blue, dark, red or yellow), suggested the cause of loss of consciousness.

*Hakim*s later monopolised the Indian medical scenario, benefitting from the patronage of the Mohammedan Princes. Diseases and remedies were divided into two classes by them – hot and cold. A hot disorder was treated by the administration of cold remedies, and *vice versa*. The concept of hot and cold treatment involved the use of drugs that either caused excessive heat in the body or produces cold – an old classification for food and drugs that has been learned and passed down through generations, and is still retained in India.

Effective interventions by the Persian *Hakim* included purging and gut-cleaning, followed by blood-letting. Then he invariably submitted his patient to natural medications, at times prescribing placebos such as syrup of violets, or sugar-candy and water. As the Persians generally had strong constitutions, they often survived; and the credit given to the physician was in direct proportion to the violence and novelty of the remedies he had employed.

A knowledgeable *Hakim* had many therapeutic secrets to cure a myriad different disorders. An anonymous surgeon published the following personal experience in the 1868 *Indian Medical Gazette*:

I was living in a malarial tract, a few years ago, where chronic spleen disease is very common and a patient, who was disappointed at my unsuccessful treatment, suddenly disappeared; but after a while, he re-appeared in my vicinity and surprised me by his altered and improved condition. His spleen was reduced to the size of a cricket ball, from having reached the umbilicus. On enquiry, I found that the sufferer had turned his back upon European science and that he had appealed successfully to the Yunani hakeem! He had taken one drop of gandhak ka tezaab (sulphuric acid) inside a bataasha or sugar bubble, every morning for a month, which he said had "cut away the congealed" mass in the organ. The man was virtually cured. ..... I have kept this old pebble in my pocket ever since, with satisfaction to myself and benefit to many an unhappy sufferer of spleen disease. It's necessary to be careful, in administering the drop, to cover the hole made in the bataasha with thick gum of flour paste.

The Christian missionaries started serving the poorer Indian population first. They spread their network deep into India. As many as 140 missionaries were working in India by 1900. Their set-up across the modern State of Chhattisgarh, served millions of tribes through schools, dispensaries and asylums. The German Evangelical Church was started in Raipur and Bishrampur towns; the American Mennonite Mission was set up in Dhamtari in 1910; and the station of the American un-sectarian establishment (called the Disciples of God), was started in Bilaspur and Mungeli. British medical services were confined to certain classes in the initial years, as noted by Col. Sleeman in his account of 1833:

All we have as yet done has been to provide medical attendants for our European officers, regiments, and jails. It must not, however, be supposed that the people of India are without medical advice, for there is not a town or considerable village in India without its practitioner (Ayurvedic/Yunani).

Gradually, confidence in English medicines and European modes of treatment, was generally established. The need for hospitals arose and they became almost as numerous as schools. India was a large experimental field for tropical diseases, and Calcutta became the principal hub for research on tropical disorders. The first medical college was started in 1835, in Calcutta.

Sir Ronald Ross worked on mosquitoes who had fed on the blood of Husein Khan, at Secunderabad, who suffered from malaria. Khan was paid one anna (6.25 paisa) per mosquito and earned 10 annas. His generous blood donation to female mosquitoes led to the discovery of the malaria parasite on 20 August 1897, otherwise known as Mosquito Day.

Haffkine (1860–1930), was a bacteriologist of Russian-Jewish descent and the first microbiologist to develop and use vaccines against cholera and plague. Haffkine moved to India in 1893, due to the poor reception of his work in the West, and remained there until his retirement in 1914. In 1896, the success of his cholera vaccine prompted the authorities to enlist him in the development of a plague vaccine, at the height of the Bombay epidemic.

Robert Koch discovered the *vibrio* organism in the stool of cholera patients in Egypt, and he later came to India. At the Medical College in Calcutta, he confirmed his discovery by finding the same *vibrio* bacilli in the stool of every cholera patient he examined in Calcutta. It took several years for bacteriologists to accept this new discovery. Some felt that Koch had displayed rather bad taste by introducing curved rather than straight bacilli.

However, the native doctors maintained that their English counterparts unable to treat chronic diseases. On the other hand, the various rules and medicines native doctors used to remove chronic fevers, was completely beyond the comprehension of the European doctors.

Among the Europeans, there were some very popular surgeons. Moreover, apart from medicine and surgery, they used their skills in several other fields as well. According to a popular story, ship surgeon Gabriel Boughton served as surgeon to the Moghul Emperor Shah Jahan, at Agra, and to his son, Shah Shuja, Governor of West Bengal in 1640–1642. He cured an imperial princess (said to be Shah Jahan's beloved, elder daughter, Jahan Ara), of a serious burn in 1636; and was instrumental in obtaining permission for initial British settlements at Hughli, near Calcutta.

In August 1715, William Hamilton, a surgeon, treated the Emperor Farrukh Siyar, for his groin swelling. Two months later, he again treated him for severe abdominal pain. In April 1717, the British were granted permission to purchase 38 villages and exempted from trade duties near Calcutta, by the Emperor.

Sir William Brooke O'Shaughnessy, Professor of Chemistry at Calcutta, was responsible for the introduction of the electric telegraph into India. He became Director General of Telegraphs at the time of the Indian Mutiny. Telegraphic communication saved India for the British Empire.

Civil Surgeons were often postmasters of the district as well, and Dr. Elijah Impey, served as Director General of the Post Office in India. Medical officers initially governed the Department of the Mint and opium production as well. Some of them contributed to the early archaeological and geographical surveys of India.

The European community had its own problems in adapting to the hot climate. Being light-coloured people used to the cold, they were negatively affected when they migrated to tropical regions. The 12 hours of daylight alternating with 12 hours of night; the invisible rays of the sun; and rainless days with stagnant air, all contributed to their *asthenia*. The term *asthenia* refers to perceived feelings of fatigue and lethargy, which can be physical (tiredness), intellectual (diminished concentration), emotional (disturbed mood) or sexual (functional sexual impotence).

The term *neurasthenia* was first used in 1879, by Dr. Beard, of New York, for a group of variable and mostly ill-defined, symptoms. Many doctors did not believe in the existence of *neurasthenia*. When a doctor could not find any specific cause for a patient's illness, it was labelled *neurasthenia*. The label *Tropical Neurasthenia*, was given to the psychological disabilities found in Europeans who lived in the tropics. Behavioural disorders were known by different names in different places (e.g. *Punjab head, Bengal head, Burmese head'* etc.). The patients suffered from headaches, sleeplessness, loss of memory, inability to concentrate, loss of emotional stability and indecisiveness – even regarding relatively unimportant matters such as whether to use a spoon or a fork. The symptoms were accompanied by increased heart rate; subnormal or unstable temperature; blood pressure on the lower side; sweating of the palms and exaggerated reflexes; dilated stomach leading to loss of appetite; and frequent mucous stools – all common physical manifestations of a state of anxiety.

For Europeans, the first year in a tropical country was particularly trying; but they learned to adapt their habits and settle down, accepting the climate as they found it in India. The Englishman grumbled in the hot weather for obvious reasons. The thought of retirement would dominate his mind unless he could find a way to get away every summer.

Not only was depression or *asthenia* common among the British, but at times, they had outbursts of anger in what was called tropical fury or fits of passion, caused by trivial incidents. This nervous irritability, the classical *furor tropicus*, of white sojourners, was undoubtedly evidence of their frustrations in adapting to local conditions.

The natives were thought to be protected from *neurasthenia* by their different lifestyle. As was often said, 'The European hustles; the native is placid'. *Neurasthenia* was, however, not uncommon among the Indian races. This complex of specific symptoms to describe depression, is common among women in Chhattisgarh, in outdoor patient units. They complain of lack of sleep, at times *tachycardia*; excessive sweating; tingling sensation in the limbs; tiredness/fatigue; backache; foul discharge per vagina; mucoid stool; and low blood pressure. Fatigue is a common symptom among women in developing countries. In one survey conducted in India, nearly a quarter of the women complained of feeling weak or tired, and more than half of them had these problems for more than six months. Fatigue in women has often been attributed to nutritional deficiencies and *anaemia*. Physicians are likely to prescribe iron, vitamins and nutritional supplements, to treat the symptom presumptively. Such preparations account for the largest category of drugs dispensed in South Asia.

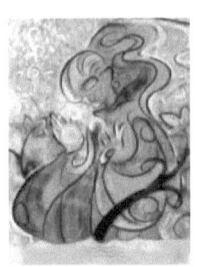

2 QUACKS, ILLNESS & SUPPORT

The following extract from a letter to the Editor of the *Hindu Patriot*, titled 'A protest against quackery of all kinds', and published in the *Indian Medical Gazette*, July 1868, provides a period picture of the rampant quackery that prevailed in the late 19th century.

...As the matter now stands, quackery knows no bounds in this country. All these classes of unprofessional men, without any knowledge of the pathology and morbid anatomy of diseases, without any attempt to ascertain their cause, or to understand their various symptoms, diagnostic, prognostic, or pathology, imprudently venture to take up the most serious cases, and, knowing the disease merely by its name, administer by turn all the medicines they have heard of in connection with the disease, without any idea of their modus operandi, or the system.

In two Asiatic medical systems, superstitious omens, lucky days, charms and religious ceremonies, were used in conjunction with traditional medicines – a practice that later generated quackery. Quacks existed even 1000 years ago in India. In Charka's essay, 'The risks of being treated by a quack', he emphasises that only a well-educated physician, approved by the association of physicians, should be allowed to treat one's person.

Niccolao Manucci was a successful European quack who benefitted from the common perception that foreigners had special knowledge of medicine. Manucci finally settled in Chennai in 1686, and then turned into a *siddha* physician. The *Siddha* system of medicine practiced in south India, is closely related to *Ayurveda*. He commented in his travel memoirs: *Not only was I famed as a doctor, but it was rumoured I had the power of expelling demons from the bodies of the possessed.*

Quacks who practice a mix of all forms of medicine, are found in large numbers across the country even today. People with little medical knowledge or skills, have found their way into society. Undoubtedly, a country that strongly believes in magic, produces more quacks than doctors. Quacks who coincidentally cure one patient, treat every other patient with precisely the same therapy, loudly trumpeting their successes while quietly burying their failures. The two main reasons behind the success of quackery across the country are the lack of qualified doctors in rural areas and the cost of medicinal services.

Henry Cayley, a surgeon posted on special duty at Ladakh, noted a very similar observation in 1867: *There are a few indigenous "medicine men" who travel about with a few drugs in a wallet and treat disease by the light of inspiration, or chance. They complain of the poverty of the land and their unrequited services.* [1]

Healers using traditional herbal medicines and rituals are scattered throughout the villages of Chhattisgarh. They have a wide reach and a flexible payment system, sometimes in kind. Illness causes instability, both socially and economically, and creates financial crisis. The people go to local quacks for the treatment of illnesses. Chicken, alcohol, rice, grain and money are spent on the same. Treatment at a Government hospital is free, but it is not available. If they visit a private doctor, the poor have to spend a great deal lot of money, which is necessarily precluded by their poverty.

In the primitive areas of Chhattisgarh, burning and branding are still used to treat pain and paralysis. It is difficult to say when and where the barbaric practices of burning and branding the skin to cure disease, started. Early European travellers to India observed

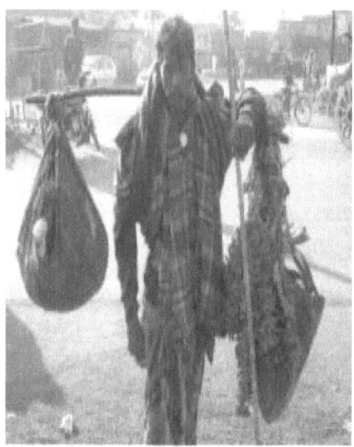 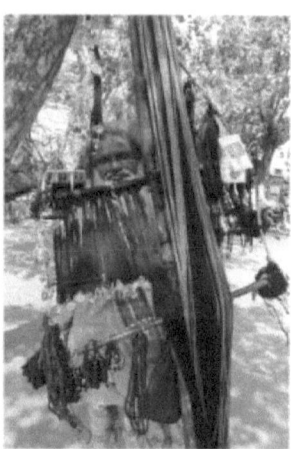

FIG 04: Left: Village drug vendor. Right: Lucky charm & sacred thread seller. Yet another group of professionals, offering their services in chronic illnesses.

these practices in the 17th century. Jean De Thevenot (1666–1667), reported the coming of skilful physicians from Kabul to India. These physicians often resorted to burning, as a part of their treatment. In Ajmer, he noted the treatment of scorpion bites with fire: *There are very venomous scorpions in that country, but Indians have several remedies to cure stinging, and best of all is fire. They take a burning coal, and apply it on the vicinity of the wound; hold it there as long and as near as they can…*

Gemelli Careri travelled to India some years later (1695–1696). He too, noted the use of burning to treat cholera (*Mordazin*) and abdominal colic (*Bornbaraki* and *Naricut*), at the port city of Daman: *Fire is also applied to the swelling (over abdomen) so that those who have the good fortune to recover carry the sign of fire afterwards on their belly.*

People in Chhattisgarh prefer conventional tattooing for aesthetic reasons and branding as a mode of treatment. Certain tribes in northern Ghana, still use scarification to treat diseases such as convulsions and tummy pains. At times, the skin is cut by a traditional healer, to deliver drugs directly into the bloodstream.

Survival with disability, even today, is even more difficult due to the lack of proper rehabilitation services. The community prefers traditional massage to physiotherapy for recovery. Recovery from stroke-related paralysis is achieved by massage. Little do they know in Chhattisgarh State, that stroke is considered to be a medical emergency! The current management of stroke requires time-based intervention. The traditional treatment is more about speedy recovery from stroke achieved by massage with castor oil and the fresh blood of a pigeon. In some places in Chhattisgarh, traditional healers use the oil of the Red Velvet mite (*Trombidium grandissimum*), also called *Birbahutti* or *Rani Keeda*, to massage paralysed limbs. The traditional healers of the Bagbahera region prepare a special oil by boiling dung beetles in mustard oil.

A smoothened, robust bamboo stick called a *lathi*, is the only walking aid available as support for villagers in cases of disability.[2] The elderly in India often walk slowly with the help of a stick in order to cope with poor vision, deformed joints, old fractures, loss of balance, and unsteadiness caused by loss of emotional confidence. In rural India, they create and conceptualise different kinds of orthotics according to their need, without the help of an occupational therapist, and learn how to carry on with crippling diseases and residual deficits. Those, who were crippled at an early age by diseases like polio, still prefer to crawl on their hands at home and on the streets. Somehow, they never adapted to the use of wheelchairs provided by governmental agencies and other charities, free of cost.

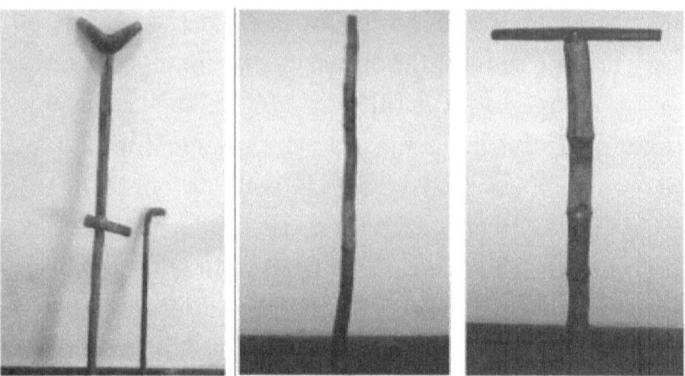

FIG 05: Walking aids – made of hardy reed and bamboo, of varying heights, a *lathi* is a simple and effective support. Disabled persons with lower limb weakness, use a *lathi* of shoulder height to jump or move forward which often resembles a mini pole vault.

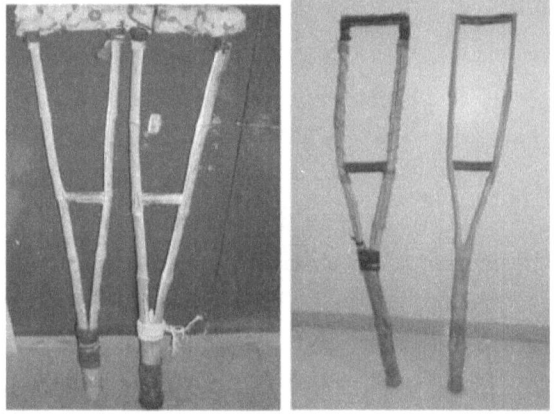

FIG 06: Homemade crutches – made by splitting a thick bamboo shaft.

Even for minor illnesses, villagers need to travel to the cities for treatment. When a villager falls ill in the interior of India, reaching a proper medical centre is a difficult task. The primary healthcare centre (PHC), is usually a few miles away, and patients are transported by any possible means. At times, the caretaker ties himself to the patient on the back seat of his motorcycle, while another person provides support to the patient by sitting on the extended carrier. Patients, who avail themselves of medical services as outpatients in the cities, start from home early in the morning and commute by share-taxi, knowing they will not return home before nightfall.

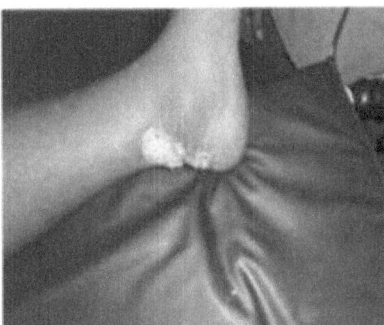 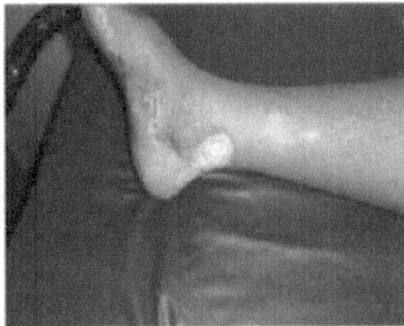

FIG 07: Woes of transportation – lesion caused by burns on the left and right feet. When BKM suffered from left-side paralysis in his village, he was transported by bike to a medical centre. Unable to balance on his own, he was sandwiched between the driver and caretaker, with his paralysed leg hanging over the muffler, so suffering burns on his inner leg. The next time, he sat facing the driver and suffered a muffler burn on his right leg.

NOTES

1. *'When the cure complete, he seeks his fee; the Devil seems less terrible than he.'*

2. *March 1830 –* 'The natives use a very dangerous weapon, which they have been forbidden by Government to carry. I took one as a curiosity, which had been seized on a man in a fight in a village. It is a very heavy lathi, a solid male bamboo, five feet five inches long, headed with iron in a most formidable manner'. Parkes, F. *Wanderings of pilgrim in search of the picturesque; Residence at Cawnpore;* 1850.

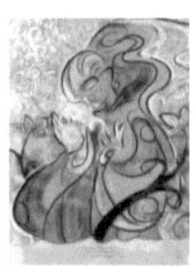

3 Epidemics, Infection & Prevention

The ancient world had its own methods of combating epidemics. Sleeman William (1788–1856), narrated a procession in the Saugar district of Central provinces, in April 1832, during an influenza epidemic. A buffalo, which had been purchased by general subscription, was driven before the noisy crowd. They were to follow it for eight miles, when it would be turned loose. If the animal returned, the disease (so it was said), would return with it. Elsewhere, a pair of scapegoats was driven to a jungle, where they were let loose; from that hour, the disease entirely ceased in the town. The goats never returned. *'Had they come back, the disease must have come back with them; so he took them a long way into the wood indeed.'*

Fanny Parkes, on 22 August 1883, noted in her diary, in Allahabad: *These natives are curious people; they have twice sent the cholera over the river, to get rid of it at Allahabad. They proceed after this fashion: they take a bull, and after having, repeated divers' prayers and ceremonies, they drive him across the Ganges into Oude laden, as they believe, with the cholera. This year, this ceremony has been twice performed. When the people drive the bull into the river, he swims across and lands, or attempts to land, on the Lucknow side; the Oude people drive the poor beast back again, when he is generally carried down by the current and drowned, as they will not allow him to land on either side.*

She also witnessed the ceremony of *Charak Puja*, to please Goddess Kali, in Calcutta, and to ward off diseases like smallpox. The deity was sought to be propitiated by men swinging from hooks: *The man*

I saw swinging looked very wild, from the quantity of opium and bhangh he had taken to deaden the sense of pain.

Bhangh is an intoxicating liquor, prepared from the leaves of the *ganja* plant (*Cannabis Indica*). The practice of *Charak Puja* is still observed, though rarely, among Hindus in Bengal and Bangladesh. Male devotees swing round in circles, suspended from a tall pole, to which they are attached with a rope and metal hooks that pierce deeply through the skin of their backs.

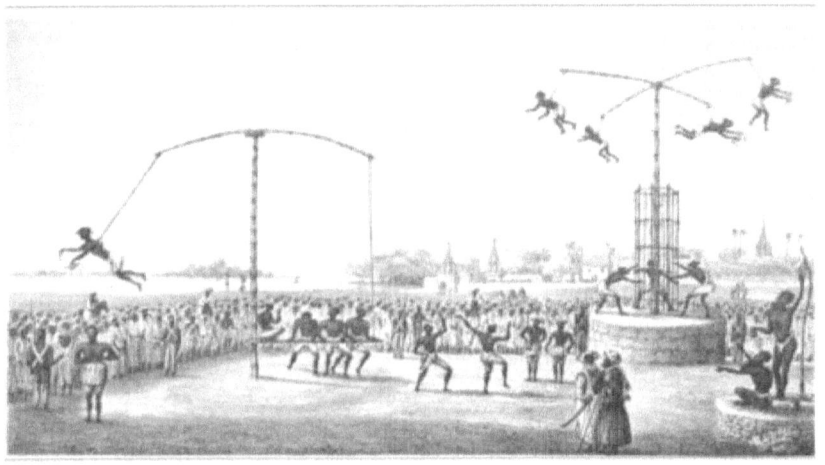

FIG 08: *Charak Puja* – a propitiatory ceremony in Bengal, featured in *Wandering of a Pilgrim in Search of the Picturesque* by Fanny Parks.

Epidemics and famine remained major killers until better strategies, drugs and a food-distribution system, came into play. Most infectious diseases would hit the country in epidemic proportions, repeatedly claiming millions of lives. Outbreaks of cholera or smallpox epidemics were common among pilgrims. In the year 1865, a pandemic of cholera, which started among the teeming thousands at the the Hindu *Kumbh Mela*, reached Bombay; and thence spread to Mecca, carried by Mohammedan pilgrims. *'The Bengal Government ordered enquiry to investigate the circumstances under which the S. S. Chollerton and S. S. Sultan were permitted to carry pilgrims under conditions which violated every law of health and which infringed the regulations of the Red Sea Pilgrim Traffic'* (Indian Pilgrims and Mecca; Nov 1893; p. 381)

A more gradual aggravation of the virulence of plague, allowed people to move out during epidemics. Because of the rather slow spread of the disease, one of the methods adopted in the countryside for prevention, was to abandon old huts and make new ones a few miles away. They would move again to a new destination if rats started dying. 'No rat-no plague' was often the call given, but the elimination of rats in Indian towns was a utopian idea that was quite incapable of fulfilment. The annual report presented by the Sanitary Commissioner, Government of India, and published in the early 1900s, cites the experience of Satara, which indicated that continuous rat trapping kept a town free from plague. That cost the Municipal Corporation one rupee per house per annum. Fortunately, plague did not reach the Raipur district in Chhattisgarh till 1903. Rats in Raipur were trapped and exposed to plague bacilli in an experiment, and they suffered 90 to 100 per cent mortality, due to lack of immunity.

The plague epidemic of 1897, caused serious havoc and people died in large numbers in Bombay and Pune. The British Government, under growing international pressure to control the disease, took stringent action to segregate the victims. Houses were searched by the military, and British troops were on the roads, to isolate plague victims. In Bombay, civilians with an army officer escort, performed this work. In Pune, this caused civil unrest against the British policy for the prevention of the spread of plague. Riots frequently broke out against the forced isolation of new arrivals by ship, to Quarantine Marine Hospital, as cholera spread from port to port. Epidemics of cholera have in the past, frequently originated at the Rajim fair site in Raipur, and also with the stream of pilgrims returning from Jagannath, Puri. In 1878 the number of deaths from cholera at Raipur was 17,000 or 20 per square mile.

During the British era, the incidence of sickness and mortality fell into three specific types. The first type included malaria, small pox, influenza, Malta fever, cerebrospinal meningitis, and typhus. The second group comprised of diseases affecting the gut –notably cholera, enteric fever, dysentery and diarrhoea. The last category consisted of lung diseases like tuberculosis, pneumonia, bronchitis etc. Most of the fatalities among European troops were caused by gut-related disorders, while native Indian troop mostly died of chest-diseases (**Appendix-2**).

The differential pattern of illness was of much interest to the scientific community. *Enteric* was another example. 60 or 70 years ago, there were many discussions in medical journals as to why *enteric* occurred among British soldiers in India, but never amongst the indigenous inhabitants; until bacteriology discovered it to be common amongst Indians. Growing awareness of microbes as the causes of disease, especially diarrhoea, reinforced the Government's concern to maintain better sanitation and the availability of clean drinking water.

The sanitary department for the prevention of smallpox, cholera and plague, carried out mass inoculation, in addition to other measures. On 10 Januar 1897, Haffkine performed the first human trial of the plague vaccine on himself. This was the first occasion a vaccine had been used on a large scale, as a public health measure and enforced by the British Government despite its adverse effects and doubtful efficacy. Figures collected by the Plague Commission suggested that this inoculation caused an 80% reduction in the infection rate and an 80 % reduction in mortality amongst those infected. Many millions of doses of this vaccine were given in India and elsewhere. In 1907, Dr Strong, working in the Philippines, used a live virulent strain of plague as a vaccine, as it had been reported that the immunity produced by this live strain was much higher than that of a dead virulent culture. This live virulent strain had been used in Java.

CONTAMINATED VACCINES ~ THE MICROBIAL FRANKENSTEIN

During the Mulkowal disaster of 1902, in which 19 Punjab villagers who had been given plague vaccine died of a tetanus contaminant – the Indian Commission reported to have *'found that the germ of tetanus had been introduced into the fluid before the bottle was opened at Mulkowal'*, and attributed the accident to laboratory operations. The Government's Plague Research Laboratory in Bombay supplied the vaccine. Waldemar Haffkine, who was in charge of the laboratory, was suspended from his post. An accidental contamination of Haffkine's anti-cholera vaccine with the plague virus, occurred in Manila in 1906. A number of natives were inoculated with the plague, and several died. It was supposed that someone placed a 48 hour virulent plague culture, insufficiently labelled, among the cholera cultures, and that the batches were mixed and inoculations immediately made.

The *Bacillus Calmette Guerin* (BCG) vaccination programme suffered a big set-back after the Lubeck disaster in 1928, when the accidental contamination of BCG with virulent tubercle bacilli, led to the deaths of 72 of 240 children vaccinated with that particular batch, in Germany.

The diseases in the tropics varied from place to place and from season to season. There was a phenomenal rise in mortality with the onset of the monsoon season. The overall trend of month-wise mortality during the British era, showed a low curve in June and reached its peak in the two subsequent months. Health was largely dependent on the climatic environment.[1]

Today, epidemics are less common (**Appendix- 3**), but there are an estimated 50 million patients suffering from infectious diseases that kill at least five million Indians every year. Central nervous system infections account for a significant number of hospital admissions; the results are promising if treatment is sought early.

NOTES

1. *People associate the occurrence of diseases with particular times of the year. During the monsoon, diarrhoea and other infectious diseases are common. Malaria is common in November and December. In the period from March to June, skin infections are common. In August and September, illnesses due to dampness are common. The monsoon is the most difficult period, as there are a number of diseases that flourish in this season and access to health services becomes difficult or even impossible, due to problems of communication and transport. Some villages become virtual islands during the rains'.* From the People; District Report, Korba Chhattisgarh Human Development Report; Government of Chhattisgarh, 2005; p. 125

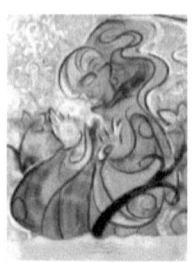

4 THE AUTUMN SCOURGE: MALARIA

The British loved to sip their favourite drink, gin mixed with Indian tonic water, while sitting on their lawns. The Indian tonic water contained a large amount of quinine dissolved in a carbonated soft drink used as a prophylactic drink against malaria. It provided a bitter taste to the gin that was preferred by British colonial India in the 1870s. Gin and tonic (Martinez) is still consumed, although tonic water now contains a much smaller amount of quinine. Apart from malaria prophylaxis sparkling aromatic quinine water was considered as a good appetizer.

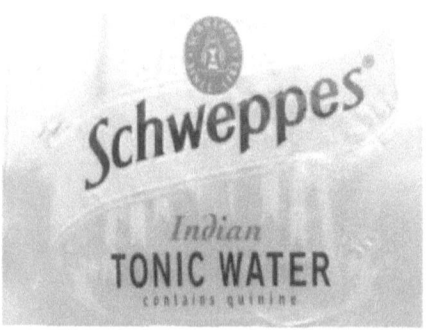

FIG 09: Indian tonic water contains a small quantity of quinine, adding a bitter taste to the gin; also thought to be useful in malaria prevention.

Malarial fever was the most frequently treated malady in hospitals during the British era, accounting for more than one-sixth of the total number of admissions. Tolerability to quinine salt was necessary for the survival of Europeans in the tropics. It was advised that all women proposing to live in the tropics be specially tested for their ability to stand quinine therapy and, if this was confirmed, they be educated to a necessary quinine standard, by regulated small doses, before being allowed to begin their new life.

THE SAGA OF CINCHONA CULTIVATION IN INDIA

Quinine became available in Europe in 1632, by way of import from Peru. The high demand for quinine, to treat intermittent fever in Europe, led to the rapid depletion of its source in Peru. The Dutch started *cinchona* cultivation in Java. The idea of cultivating *cinchonas* on the Indian subcontinent was first considered by Dr. Royale, who obtained some plants from various botanical gardens in Great Britain. Five of these plants reached Calcutta alive but did not thrive in the Royal Botanic Gardens on the banks of the Hooghly. Thus, they were transferred to Darjeeling. Only three survived the transit. On 14 May 14 1855, Dr Campbell, the Superintendent of Darjeeling, stated: *'[A]ll the three cinchona trees were killed by the cold of last winter'*.

The Markham expedition is a remarkable episode in the history of *cinchona* importation. On 5 April 1859, Clements Markham, in a communication to Sir George Clerk, volunteered to go out to South America for the purpose of securing introduction of *cinchona* plants into India. The choice of Markham for this mission was perfect, as a few years earlier he had travelled through Peru extensively. Markham, accompanied by his wife and accomplished botanist Richard Spruce, arrived in Lima in January of 1860. When ready, the party set out on an expedition over high and rough paths and roads. They reached Apo, a village 14,350 feet above sea level. Most of the party and even the transport animals, suffered from mountain sickness. They continued until they reached the huge Lake Titicaca, and then they entered into the forests of Caravaya. But the object of the expedition came under some suspicion by the Peruvian authorities, causing all sorts of obstacles to be placed in his way. Despite many difficulties, including scarcity of food, he succeeded in ultimately bringing numerous plants down to the seacoast port of Islay on 9 June 1860, including 456 of the more valuable species. On 28 July, he met with further difficulties from the customs authorities; but Markham managed to obtain a government permit and get the plants on board the ship, just in time to escape an attempt to destroy the plants by pouring boiling water on them. He reached Southampton with the Wardian cases containing the collection of plants, which were, overall, in good condition. More than 216 plants had begun to throw out shoots.

On 27 August 1860, Markham sailed for India, touching Bombay and Calicut, with the stock in hand. He reached Ootacamund on 12 October, with all the cases containing the *Calisayan* species of *cinchona*. Markham's larger consignments were not so fortunate. They were shipped to India in September, through the heat of the Red Sea. They were further detained in Bombay for a week, and when they reached the Nilgiris, they were dying. On 26 February, Markham reported that his earlier expectations of the final recovery of the plants, which had arrived in the 'Neilgherry' Hills the previous October, had been disappointed, and that he was *'unable to entertain hopes of the ultimate recovery of more than one'*. Even this last one perished despite all Markham's care and personal attention.

Cinchona was later grown successfully in the hills of Darjeeling and Nilgiri, with seeds and plants brought by Mr Cross from Kew and Dr Anderson from Java. In Sri Lanka, it was planted around1861 in the Hakgala Botanical Gardens at Nuwara Eliya and were looked after by James Taylor.

The *cinchona* tree grows slowly; it takes about eight years before any yield can be expected, and much longer before this yield reaches its maximum. Among the variant species of *cinchona* that were cultivated, were those with red bark, yellow bark and crown bark. The bark alkaloids included *quinine, quinidine, cinchonine, cinchonidine* and sometimes *arecin*. All alkaloids were considered efficacious in curing fever, but the yellow bark yielded quinine of superior quality. The specialist who looked after quinine production was known as a quinologist.

Quinologist C.H. Wood, prepared a non-crystalline extract of the bark. This was a yellowish powder composed of a mixture of the alkaloids exclusively derived from the red-bark trees (*C. Succirubra*). It was named *cinchona febrifuge* (*totaquina*). Over the next 12years, this febrifuge continued to be the sole manufactured product of the factory in Bengal. The unfortunate impression that gained ground relating to *cinchona* febrifuge, was that it was a cheap and inferior substitute for quinine. One of the reasons for the unpopularity of the *totaquina* as a preparation was the lack of standards in such mixtures.

INGENUITY IN QUININE DISTRIBUTION

Efforts were, however, continued to extract quinine but for a long time the trade secrets were zealously guarded in England and Germany. At long last in 1888, J. Gemmie, succeeded in making quinine in Bengal and its use was soon widespread in India.

In 1892, at the instance of the Bengal Government, the post office began acting as an agency for the sale of quinine produced at the government factory. This measure was introduced tentatively, and the drug was placed on sale at post offices in five-grain powders at a quarter of an anna (1.56 paisa). Upon the experiment proving successful, it was gradually extended to the whole of India. Between 1903 and 1904, more than seven million packets were sold in this way. Bengal was later accused of making a handsome profit out of the cultivation, manufacture and sale of quinine. In the Central Provinces, quinine and *cinchona* preparations were supplied from the Central Jail, Nagpur. The system of retailing packets of quinine through the post office, was introduced in the Central Provinces in 1893. Besides postmasters, the services of school masters, stamp-vendors, and *patwaris*, were occasionally utilised as drug vendors. The cultivation of *cinchona* flourished for some years in India and Ceylon until, in the year 1887, Ceylon alone produced 16 million pounds of *cinchona* bark. The British government failed to keep pace with the Dutch planters in Java due to a lack of political will; and India soon lost out in the competition for the world market, and Java acquired a complete monopoly. About 70,000 pounds of *cinchona* alkaloids, of which quinine formed the bulk, were produced in India annually, while the average amount consumed was 200,000 pounds. By the 1940s, the balance requirement had to be imported from Java.

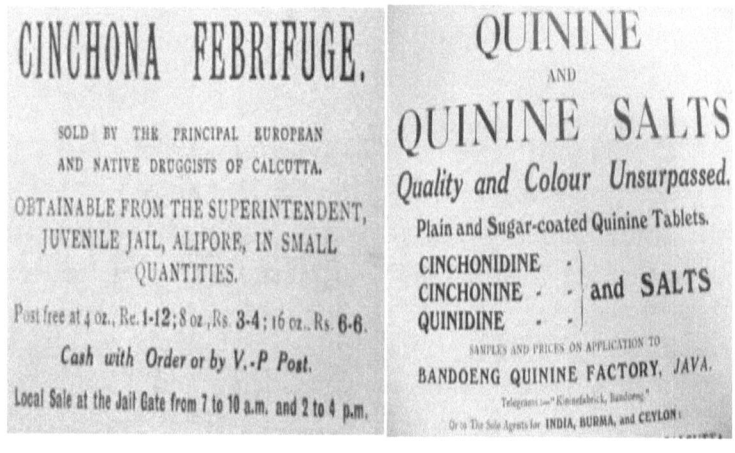

FIG 10: **Sale of *cinchona* febrifuge** at jail gates in Bengal and imported quinine from Java.

THE ONGOING CRUSADE AGAINST MALARIA

One of the chief destroyers of life and health in India is still malaria. Importantly, there is a seasonal pattern to the malarial menace in that deaths from the disease normally peaks during the autumn months. People attribute this high autumnal incidence of malarial death to the influence of the autumn moon. Malaria is endemic in the tribal-dominated regions of the peninsular states, including Chhattisgarh,

> For over 120 years the finest Quinine has been made by Howards of Ilford. The present shortage of supplies is due to enemy action but we hope before long to again supply our friends with all their requirements of Quinine, of the traditional Howards' quality.

FIG 11: An acute shortage of quinine occurred during World War II, when Java was occupied by the Japanese.

which has as many as seven malaria-prone districts owing to heavy rainfall and its dense forests. Cases are seen throughout the year in jungles, but there are significantly more between August and December. After its near-eradication in the early and mid-1960s, with the massive use of insecticides (especially DDT), malaria is now back. Mosquitoes have now developed resistance to DDT, and the plasmodium parasite is resistant to quinine. As a result, we are now fighting a full-fledged chemical war against mosquitoes in our homes, using *prallethrin* (All-out), *d-trans allethrin* (Hit) etc.; and on streets with intensive supervised spraying.

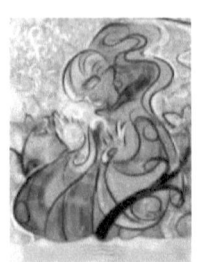

5 AFFLICTIONS ON THE WANE – SYPHILIS & YAWS

The absence of general paralysis among the insanity cases from the Indian asylums is rather interesting. It is, however, in accordance with global experience. In the authoritative words of Savage (*Allbutt's System, Vol. VII*, p. 693): *[G]eneral paralysis is rare among vegetable feeders, such as certain Oriental races, though these may give way to excessive sexual indulgence. I understand that certain nomadic tribes, though saturated with syphilis, not being addicted to meat nor alcohol, do not get general paralysis... The disease is associated with highly civilised States and most common among men who live in cities and do brain work. Diabetes in some respects takes the place of general paralysis among educated city-dwelling natives of India.*
~ Insanity in India; Indian Medical Gazette, October 1899

SYPHILIS
Syphilis is a venereal disease caused by an infection from the bacteria *Treponema pallidum*. Syphilis was first introduced to north India almost 500 years ago. The disease spread through land routes to the hilly areas of Afghanistan, Nepal, Baluchistan and Shimla, chiefly via the invading armies. Portuguese sailors spread syphilis around the Port of Calicut and also infected women with the dreaded disease of the Great Pox. In 1895, the disease attacked the British troops in India on an unprecedented scale – almost half the hospital admissions were due to some form of the disease. The ratio of admission was 511 per 1000 in 1896 and 507.8 in 1897. Taking the mean of three years, the ratios of admission per 1000,

due to the disease in Europe and Asia, were as follows: Germany 27.3; Russia 43.0; France 43.8; Great Britain 203.7; and India 438.0.

For every 100 hospital admissions during the British-Raj (1895–1899), the incidence of venereal disease was much higher among British-European troops as compared to native soldiers (**Appendix-6**). British soldiers were permitted to visit prostitutes although such indulgences were prohibited for the higher ranked officers. The first major concern of the British Raj in India regarding Indian women's welfare, was to eliminate venereal disease, since it became a serious problem in the army. Army cantonments had officially sanctioned brothels which were disease-free. The only way to control the spread of the disease was to quarantine prostitutes who were infected, until they recovered in a hospital. The necessity for the 'lock hospital' arose from The Contagious Disease Act for the Prevention of Venereal Disease, passed by the legislature.[1] The prevention of venereal disease was intimately connected to the control of prostitution by the police department. The Act required the compulsory registration of prostitutes; compulsory periodical medical examinations of prostitutes; and the compulsory detention of diseased prostitutes in 'lock hospitals' until they were certified as cured. A report from the Commissioner of Police, published in the 1860s, registered the number of common prostitutes in Calcutta at about 6,000.

Prophylaxis against syphilis was seriously considered in the Indian Army through syphilisation – a method introduced by Auzias-Turenne of Paris. The method involved repeated inoculations of the syphilitic matter taken from primary sores, sometimes with as many as 250 punctures in the body. Such prophylactic efforts were, however, soon given up due to proven failure in a number of inoculated persons. Apart from Chinese root (*Sarsaparilla*), heavy metals like arsenic, bismuth, bromides and mercurous chloride (calomel), were used frequently in hopes of 'burning' away the disease.

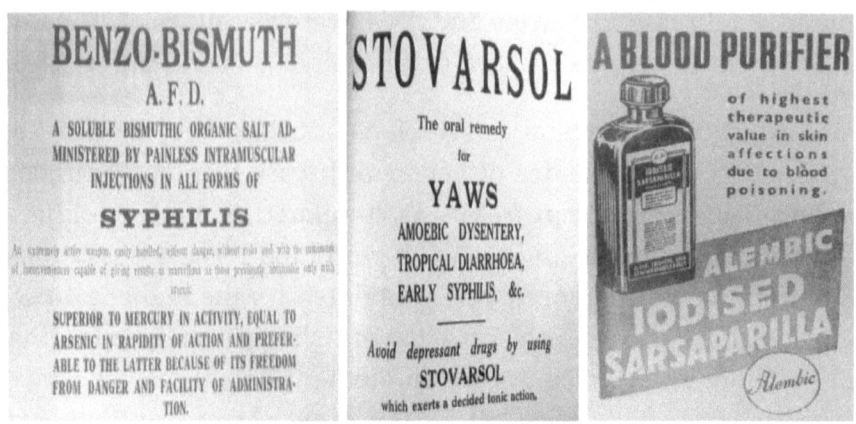

FIG 12: Sexually transmitted diseases: Syphilis was often treated with heavy metals like arsenic and mercury before the availability of penicillin. Another preparation of arsenic (*Acetarsone*), was applied in treating yaws and congenital syphilis. Chinese root (*sarsaparilla*), was also introduced as a treatment for syphilis.

Neuro-syphilis has become an infrequently reported disease in recent times. There were no cases of advanced syphilis causing dementia, at the famous Mayo Clinic (USA), from 1990 to 1994. The gradual decline in its incidence was also reported in African countries such as Morocco and Kenya. However, after decades of decline, the rate of primary and secondary syphilis has again begun to register an upsurge in association with HIV. In the state of Chhattisgarh, the disease still persists and lunatic and demented syphilitic patients are referred from the psychiatric unit. Ten cases of neuro-syphilis have been identified in the recent past. All the patients had HIV-negative status, and five patients had progressive dementia with prominent psychiatric symptoms and rigid posturing. None improved, owing to the advanced state of the disease. In the past, all inmates of mental asylums worldwide were periodically screened for syphilis but is now a forgotten practice. This has resulted in a number of cases being left undiagnosed.

In 1920, all the inmates of the Ranchi European Lunatic Asylum, who hailed from northern, central, and eastern India, were examined by Major Owen Berkeley-Hill, using the Wassermann syphilis reaction test. In all, 186 individuals were tested, 73 reacted positively, and 113 reacted negatively, thereby indicating a percentage of latent syphilis to the extent of 39.24 % of the total asylum population.

YAWS

There was a Ceylon connection to the research breakthroughs with regard to the causative agents behind both syphilis and yaws. Aldo Castellani was appointed to the Central Laboratory in Colombo in 1903. Soon after the discovery that spirochetes caused syphilis, by Schaudinn, he discovered, while working in Ceylon, the organism responsible for the treponemal disease called Yaws.

Yaws was endemic in most of the tribal districts of Chhattisgarh. Of the 16 districts, 13 reported Yaws cases, with Bastar district reporting the highest number. Yaws is caused by a treponemal subspecies called *pertenue*. It mainly affects the skin and bones (through ulceration), and it is not a sexually transmitted disease. People affected with the disease often ignore initial skin lesions, and in the later stages, cannot walk to the nearest healthcare centre due to pain and ulcers in the legs. Yaws was first noticed in India in 1887, among the tea plantation workers of Cachar district in Assam. Yaws became endemic in several parts of the country during the 1940s, especially in the geographically contiguous stretch in Chhattisgarh which included Sarguja, Bastar and Bilaspur districts.

India implemented the Yaws Control Programme from 1952 to 1964 (involving penicillin injections), with support from the WHO and other international agencies, which greatly reduced the number of cases. The country reportedly reached 'nil' new case status in 2004. An expert group meeting was held on 20 April 2006, under the chairmanship of Dr S. Pattanayak, Former Regional Advisor, World Health Organization, to discuss the status of elimination.

Subsequently, the fifth Task Force Meeting was held on 31 May 2006, and a 'declaration of elimination' was recommended.

Notwithstanding the official position based on the absence of new case findings, it needs to be borne in mind that the disease affected the marginalised population residing in the remote tribal belt of Chhattisgarh. In most of the tribal areas which were endemically afflicted by Yaws, the posts of Medical Officers lay vacant. The region was also the worst affected by an upsurge in Maoist activity. Hence, it is difficult to validate the claim that the disease has been eliminated from such remote and inaccessible corners of the state.

NOTES

1. *'It was counted impious that bazaar prostitutes should be inspected or that the men be taught elementary precautions in dealing with them. This official virtue cost our Army in India nine thousand expensive white men a year laid up with venereal disease'.* Rudyard Kipling: *Something of Myself.*

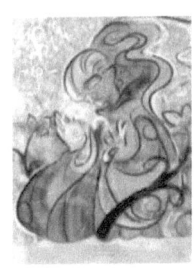

6 THE PERCEIVED CURSE: LEPROSY

The diseases named below are transmitted from one person to another by sexual intercourse, by touch, by the breath, by sharing meals in the same dish, by sleeping on the same bed and sitting on the same seat, by sharing same garments, by wearing the same garland and by sharing ointments: leprosy, fever, consumption, ophthalmia and smallpox of different kinds.
[Susruta, *The ancient and leprosy; Indian Medical Gazette*: Nov 1893.]

Leprosy has existed in India, Ceylon and Burma for centuries, without substantial spread. In India, it is confined to a certain region including the state of Chhattisgarh. The first mention of leprosy is found in the ancient Vedic Indian treatise written in the early days of the Indus Valley civilisation. The disease was also part of folklore and mythology and legend. Alberuni, a Persian scholar who visited India around 1017 AD, narrated a mythical story: Fire disturbed Lord *Shiva* while the deity was cohabiting with his divine consort; consequently, Lord *Shiva* cursed Fire with the disease of leprosy. On being thus afflicted, Fire felt so ashamed that it plunged deep into the Earth. As the gods missed Fire, they went in search for it. When the divinities finally found Fire, it refused to join them, because it was leprous. The gods restored it to health and freed it from leprosy. They brought Fire back and made it the mediator between God and humankind. According to Indian mythology, offering human sacrifices to please another Vedic God, *Varuna*, can cure leprosy.

According to still another legend, Lord *Krishna*, angered by his son *Shamva*'s apparent act of impropriety, cursed him with leprosy. In a bid to mitigate its effect, *Shamva* was directed to propitiate *Surya* (the Sun god), the healer of all skin diseases. Following 12 years of severe penance, he succeeded in pleasing the god and was cured of his illness. In gratitude, Shamva decided to erect a temple in honour of *Surya*, at *Konark* (the famous Sun Temple). The sight of impoverished lepers wandering about and displaying the ravages of the disease for the purpose of evoking charity, is common in India. Even today, lepers gather outside the Sun Temple and other religious places and sit in line for food and help. The superstitious say that for such an ugly disease to affect human beings, it must be the result of a sin committed in the past. Some even believe that leprosy results from the murder of *brahmins*, women and virtuous men; theft; or adultery (recent or during past lives).

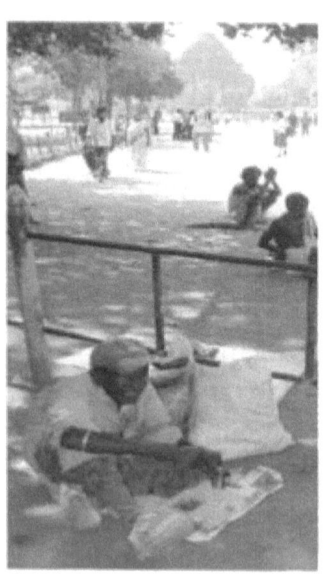

FIG 13: Curse & Cure. Lepromatous patient sitting opposite the Sun Temple *Konark* (Courtesy: Ram Mohan Bajpai)

HOLY WATER BATH

A dip in a holy water pond was thought to wash away all sins and also believed to cure leprosy and other skin diseases. From ancient times, sufferers in search of a cure for their leprosy, have often visited such sacred ponds. According to the *Imperial Gazetteer* of India, in the early 1900s, many such holy sites existed across the country. For example, *Padma Tirtha* in *Basim* (Akola district); Unnao (near Datia), Bhongaon in the Mainpuri district of the United

Provinces; *Mandargiri* in the Bhagalpur district of eastern India; Tarn Taran in Punjab (north India); and *Pakshitirtham*, Tirukkalikkunram, in south India, were all famous as spots for lepromatous to take a dip in the holy waters.

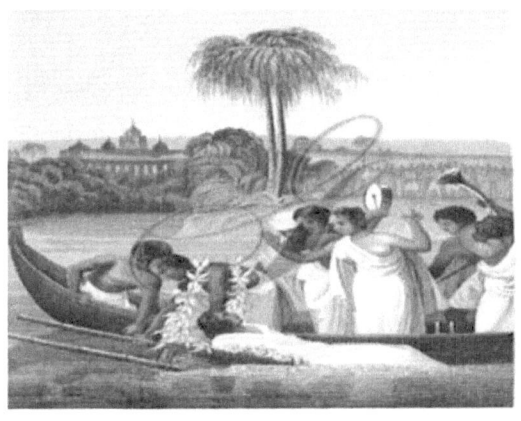

FIG 14: Drowning of lepromatous patient in south India during bathing in holy pond (courtesy of Granger collection New York).

SEARCH FOR CAUSALITY: ROTTEN FISH & RAINFALL

Jonathan Hutchinson, a British scientist, documented the origin of the disease in fish and its transmission to humans via the consumption of rotten fish. The high prevalence of the disease in the coastal states was advanced in support of the theory. Rumours were rife among the scientific community regarding the growth of the causative organism for leprosy in fish broth. Jonathan Hutchinson visited Calcutta in 1901, in search of more evidence to support his theory of fish causing leprosy. However, India disappointed him, as there was little evidence to validate his theory. For example, in the Punjab, there were 113 lepers in the Leper Asylum at Tarn Taran. Of those, 77 had never consumed fish, 6 seldom ate fish and 30 did so regularly. However, as he recalled in his publication, he found support for the theory in Ceylon: *A man, recently returned from Ceylon, tells me that there, the disease is generally ascribed to the eating of rotten fish, which the natives curry and eat freely.*

The Leprosy Commission in India, however, rejected Hutchinson's fish theory. The Commissioners found over 50 lepers whose principles enforced abstinence from fish. Even so, word spread through the missionaries and those with leprosy at Chhattisgarh stopped consuming fish.

In 1923, Sir Rogers published maps showing a close worldwide relationship between high rainfall and high incidence of leprosy. He stressed his point using the leprosy census figures and a study of rainfall records across India. The only exception was that the disease appeared to have spread from the Bombay coast into the comparatively dry Deccan, along the oldest trade routes in India.

OIL FOR TREATMENT

Various oils were commonly used in India to treat leprosy. *Unnao* treatment (*ichthyol* and *resorcin*), recommended by the Indian Government, was largely unsuccessful. However, Madar (*calotropis gigantea*) and Asiatic Pennywort (*hydrocotyle asiatica*), two common Indian plants, attained a considerable reputation in the treatment of leprosy.

Chandkhuri was an important mission centre at Chhattisgarh and had a large leper asylum. Dr Milton C. Lang, Medical Superintendent of the Chandkuri Asylum, in his annual report for 1926, summarised the results of the quarterly examinations of the in-patients at the asylum. He reported an average of 183 patients as having undergone treatment for a whole year, receiving two injections weekly of either pure *hydnocarpus* oil with *creosote* and *olive* oil, or the diluted esters of *hydnocarpus* oil. Of these patients, an average of 85 showed improvement, 69 remained the same and 29 became worse.

Chaulmoogra oil was used to treat leprosy in northeast India, China and Burma, as a folk medicine. The fruit and seeds of the *chaulmoogra* tree (*hydnocarpus*) were part of Burmese folklore, Indian mythology and Ayurvedic legacy. Frederic John Mouat of the Indian Medical Service, first used the oil in modern medicine. While the *cinchona* tree and its seeds were brought to India, *chaulmoogra* was exported to various corners of the world. In 1920, an adventurous botanist, Joseph Rock, visited Singapore in search of the tree. He was aware of the existence of the *chaulmoogra* tree but unaware of its appearance and location. To find it, he explored the eastern jungles. Finally, he found seeds for sale in a native Indian market. The seeds were collected and taken to America. In 1921–1922, 980 trees were planted on the island of Oahu in Hawaii. Subsequently, however, use of the oil was replaced with effective sulfones in the 1940s.

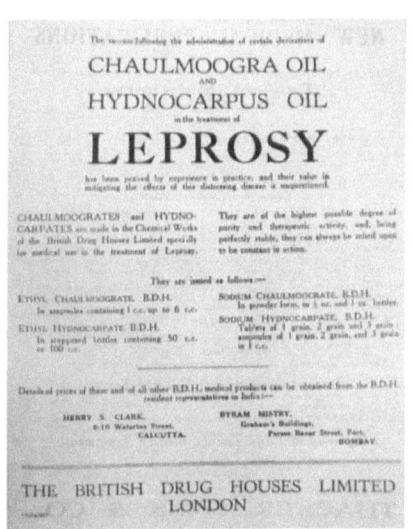

FIG 15: **Leprosy treatment** – massage with *hydnocarpus* and *chaulmoogra* oils.

Leper asylums were maintained in a number of places in Chhattisgarh by missionaries, in order to segregate and treat lepers. The asylums did sterling service to people afflicted with leprosy. Some of the priests and nuns devoted their entire lives to the mission.

As per governmental claims, the country achieved the goal of eradicating leprosy in December 2005. However, despite the constant denial by government agencies that it still exists, leprosy is seen quite often in our medical practice. Chhattisgarh is one of the three states yet to achieve the goal of elimination. Between 2008 and 2009, 7994 new cases were registered in the Chhattisgarh state records. In fact, the prevalence has remained the same (about seven – five males and two females – per 10,000 people), since the earlier British survey. In most parts of India, the milder neural form of the disease predominates, in which the nerves are thickened with or without subtle skin patches, along with blunted sensation, unlike in its more destructive form.

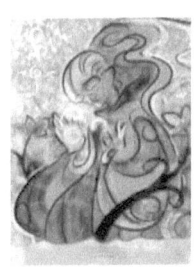

7 LIVING IN HOPE: TUBERCULOSIS

Dr Kennedy had noticed a similar "most remarkable increase" amongst the aboriginal tribes in Chota Nagpur, and this, he attributed to the growing practice for the men to go to work as coolies in Calcutta or in the Bengal coal mines . . . It is commonly recognised that young people travelled from Central India or the Deccan to work or study in Bombay or the "Konkan" involves a definite measure of risk of consumption...
[Lankester, A. *Tuberculosis in India: Its prevalence, causation & prevention*; 1920]

In the 20th century, tuberculosis (TB) spread through the country like wildfire. The need for TB dispensaries, hospitals, wards and sanatoria was felt throughout the country. TB sanatoria were situated in hill stations and other beautiful locations. The first Indian open-air sanatorium was established in Tilounia in Ajmer; and very soon, sanatoria with reputations for the successful treatment of TB were established across the country. A small institution for Christian women and girls opened in Pendra, near Bilaspur in Chhattisgarh, a small hill station situated in the Satpura mountains, on the Bombay-Howrah rail route. The affluent class was treated in exotic locations in Europe, mostly at sanatoria located in Switzerland.

No effective medication was available to treat TB in earlier times, and the backbone of sanatorium treatment was merely fresh air, good food and other hygienic measures. Among the remedies used were injections of various heavy-metal salts and calcium as well as auto-vaccines. In terms of survival before the advent of modern anti-tubercular drugs, Madanapalle, a Union Mission TB sanatorium in south India, recorded in 1916 and 1925, a low survival rate for advanced cases of the disease. (**Appendix-4**)

Encouraged by the success achieved by the experiments of McFadyean and Von Behring in immunising cattle against TB, it was decided to extend this experiment to human beings. For general application, it was necessary to employ live cultures, though with much lower virulence.

Two French scientists invented BCG. Calmette took a virulent bovine strain of mycobacterium TB, which, on repeated sub-cultures every three weeks, gradually lost its virulence. Calmette further attenuated this strain by 230 serial sub-cultures between 1908 and 1921. The original strain of BCG has been lost and has been replaced by a variant at the Pasteur Institute. In India, the BCG Vaccine Laboratory was started in 1948, in Guindy, Madras. The Danish strain 1331, was used for the preparation of both liquid and freeze-dried vaccines, based on the 'seed lot' system.

After a pilot trial in Madanapalle in 1948, where the modalities of a mass BCG drive were worked out, the Indian BCG campaign was launched in 1951. In general, the extent of vaccination across the country now is very good. As per the various surveys, BCG coverage in the state of Chhattisgarh is around 74.3 %. BCG helps prevent the disease spreading through the blood. In children, vaccination shows a better protective effect against the infiltration of the brain covering (tuberculous meningitis) and fine mottling of the lung (miliary TB). However, the efficacy of the vaccine reduces closer to the equator, and the protective effect of BCG against TB is modest in India (at best 30% to 50%). The largest community-based controlled trial of the BCG vaccination was conducted from 1968 to 1971, in south India. No protective efficacy in either adults or children was demonstrated five years after vaccination. The recently conducted meta-analyses also reveals that it is not useful in preventing pulmonary or extra-pulmonary TB in adolescents and adults. The effectiveness of BCG vaccinations to protect against TB is now under scrutiny.

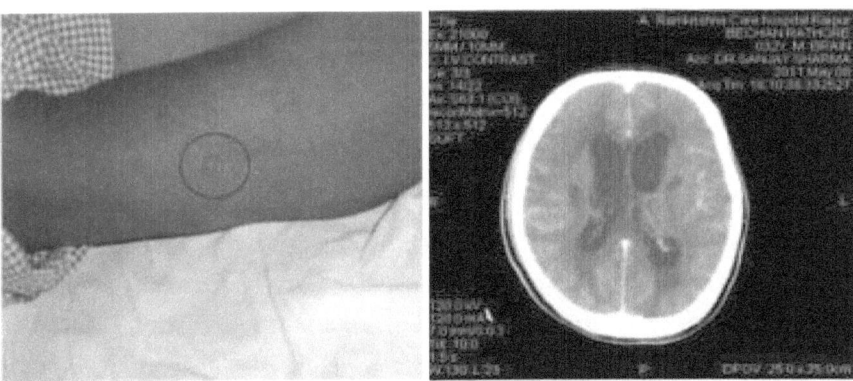

FIG 16: Failed vaccination. Advanced tubercular inflammation of the brain in a young BCG-vaccinated male. Good mark on the arm indicates an effective vaccination (encircled).

Tubercular meningitis, tuberculoma and spinal TB, are commonly seen in the advanced stages of the disease, with patients travelling to hospitals from remote places for treatment. The brain fills with tubercular exudate, like a white sauce, or tiny nodules of tuberculoma, that spread all over the craniospinal axis; the vertebrae are eaten up by the TB disease, and sometimes fine miliary tubercles fill up the lungs and brain simultaneously. Anti-tubercular drugs have many adverse effects and need to be taken over extended periods. The inability of patients to tolerate the anti-tubercular medicines leads to the frequent discontinuation of therapy. To further complicate matters, tubercular bacilli are becoming resistant to standard anti-tubercular medication.

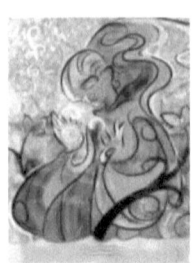

8 Worms in the Gut & Brain: Neurocysticercosis

Convulsions and nervous affections occurring in Natives and Anglo-Indians are very frequently due to the presence of worms in the intestines. Their existence may perhaps be unsuspected or even denied. Hence, in all cases which resist ordinary treatment, it is advisable to give a trial to one or more of the remedies recommended for worms, especially those for the lubricous or round worm, which is so extensively prevalent in India. [Waring, E.J. *Remarks on the uses of the bazaar medicines and common medical plants of India*, 1883]

Cysticercosis, a larval tapeworm infection, is transmitted to humans through pigs. While infected meat remains a valid explanation for its spread in humans, the mode of transmission among the vegetarian population is still not clear. An inspection of slaughterhouses in the north revealed pork meat infested with *cysticerci larvae*. The parasitized meat was called 'measly pork'. One of the problems which persist is the killing of pigs outside the slaughterhouse, as it is prohibited to kill pigs in slaughterhouses in India for religious reasons (as is the case with the holy cow). Hence, official inspections of such meat have never been conducted.

J. Flemming reported that 2651 cattle were slaughtered during the year 1868, for the use of troops and of this number, 235 (8.86%), were found to be infected with cysts. The following year, in January 1869, 367 were slaughtered and 125 were found to be cyst infected (37.09%), and for the month of February, 381 were slaughtered and 101 condemned for the same reason (27.29%).

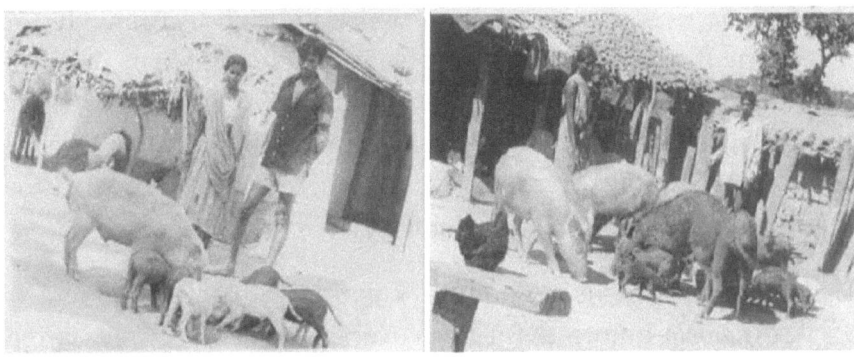

FIG 17: Pig farming in tribal regions of Chhattisgarh.

Ayurveda identified six types of gut worms residing in the rectum as also five types of bloodworms. Many plants with anthelmintic properties were identified. These plant preparations either directly or indirectly kill or render powerless and expel, intestinal parasites from the alimentary canal.

Specific tapeworm-killer herbal medications have been described in earlier literature. *Arecoline*, an active ingredient of betel nut which is regularly chewed by Indians, was found to be an effective tapeworm killer. The male fern was one of the oldest and most potent medications for tapeworm infestation; during the Greco-Roman period, it was recommended for expelling tapeworm. Louis XVI of France paid a huge sum to obtain a formula containing this drug. A mixture of a male fern plant resin and an essential oil (*oleoresin*), was used for many years until more effective medications became available. The Abyssinians were fond of raw beef, and the Chinese loved their opium, both of which caused tapeworm infestations in the gut. *Kousso (Bragira anthelmintica)*, an Abyssinian tree found in the mountains at over 10,000 feet, was the national remedy for tapeworm, and each dose was taken once a month (Extracts, IMG, 1869).

The *Embella ribes (Baberang)* plant was also used as a remedy for tapeworm. It was also called 'false black pepper' due to its pungent pepper-like taste. James Irving was the first to publish on the utility of the drug (found in Indian bazaars), in IMG (1869). However, it was an article by Dr Harris in the *Lancet* (1887), that attracted the attention of the scientific community.

Mallotus philippensis is a plant of the spurge family. It is known as the *Red Kamala* due to the fruit's covering, which produces a red dye. *Kamala*, often employed by the natives as a dye in earlier times, was also available in the form of a beautiful purple-red powder. In medicine, it had considerable repute as a remedy for Taenia tapeworm but was known to have little or no effect on other forms of intestinal worms. The dose for an adult was two to three drachms in honey or a little aromatic water, with no other medicine before or after. This dosage acted freely on the bowels, causing in many instances, considerable nausea and abdominal pain. The worm was generally expelled in a lifeless state in the third or fourth stool. If the first intake did not prove successful, the dose was typically repeated after a week.

The root-bark of the pomegranate tree was a remedy of established value for tapeworm. The fresh bark was sliced and boiled in water which was drunk in the morning in a fasting state and repeated every half-hour until four doses had been taken. This was followed by one ounce of castor oil. The worm was generally expelled within 12 hours. The root-bark of the male tree was supposed to possess the greatest power in such cases.

Cysticercosis is a common parasitic disease, and at times it reaches the brain. It is the main cause of acquired epilepsy in developing countries. Neuro-cysticercosis was documented in large numbers among the British military but rarely reported in Indian natives, perhaps due to different eating habits.

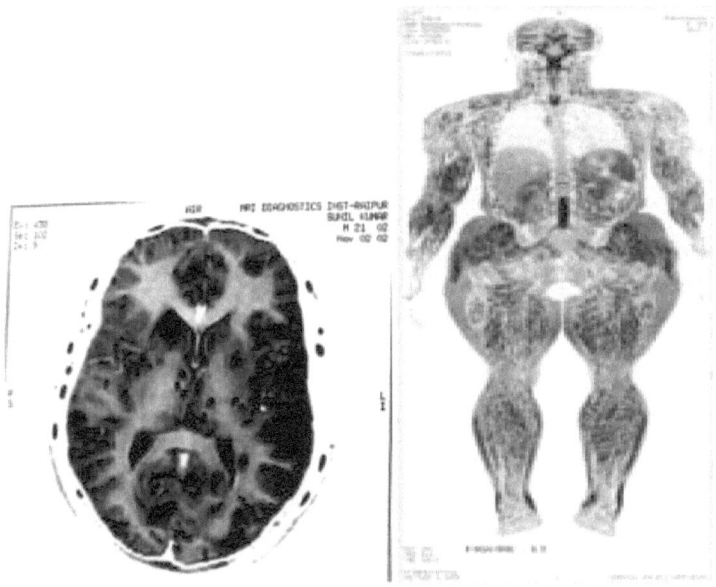

FIG 18: Florid distribution of cysticerci in the human body. The lack of muscle space free of the parasite, and presence of cysts in the scalp, always suggest widespread dissemination. Case: A 23-year-old female was admitted with features of raised intracranial tension and low-grade fever of two months duration. She had experienced two episodes of generalised convulsion. An examination showed bulging calf muscles and pea-sized palpable nodules beneath the skin. Her MRI revealed disseminated cysticercosis involving the brain parenchyma and a massive infiltration of the skeletal muscle. She died six months later.

The first Indian record of cysticercosis was an autopsy report by Surgeon H. Armstrong in 1888. He described a case of *cysticercus cellulosae* of the brain in a native cooly, aged 33 years, who had been sent to the Madras Asylum as a criminal lunatic from Nellore Jail. The patient died of exhaustion from epileptiform fits. An autopsy revealed *cysticercus granuloma* in the brain, and incidentally, he also had cardiac cysts.

Williams (1906), described the dissemination of the disease to the tongue. Later on, George R. McRobert (1944), reported nodular infiltration of the *masseter* muscle responsible for jaw clenching. And Colonel Johnson noted *temporalis* muscle *cysticerci* in an exploratory operation.

Infective larvae sometimes invade muscles throughout the body, leaving not even a centimetre of free space, leading to the Herculean enlargement of muscles. The presence of cysts in the eyes, tongue and salivary glands and beneath the skin, all suggests a disseminated disease.

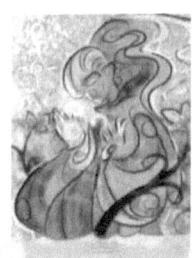

9 FUNGUS

The irresistible urge to rub the groin many times a day, is a constant source of embarrassment for many. The agent that causes the irritation is a fungus popularly known as ringworm. The condition was also a matter of concern for the men of the British Army, while in uniform. In the army, the problem was said to have resulted from bad laundering: *The dhobis would bring back your shirts ironed with knife-edge creases. It is likely that the seams inside were stiff with starch, and this resulted in the itch.*

Indian washermen were blamed for the problem and it was known as *dhobi* itch. Some scientists also laid the blame at the washermen's door, as mentioned in Napier: *The popular tradition (undoubtedly founded on facts) that the dhobi or Indian washer-man, before returning to their owner the clothes he has taken home to wash, lends or hires them out to his friends, whose mycotic infections are thus widely disseminated.* [1, 2]

Little did scientist, soldier and layperson alike, know that the problem was actually a *fungus* which caused the *dhobi* itch. In 1844, Gruby first suggested that ringworm was due to a parasitic fungus. Castellani cultured the responsible fungus and identified it as *epidermophyton cruris*. [Castellani & Chalmers, Manual of Tropical Medicine, 1910]

The *Arthashastra* lays down the following rules: *Washermen and tailors shall not wear, sell, hire out, mortgage, lose or change a customer's garment. They shall return the garments within the time prescribed.*

A stringent financial punishment (12 coins), was applied to washermen found guilty of leasing out clothes.

Scattered patches of *tinea* infection over the inner thigh and elsewhere on the body, as well as fungus growth in the nasal sinuses and the space behind the orbit, from *rhinosporidiosis* and *aspergilloma*, are acquired mostly from bathing in dirty village ponds with immune-competent and immune-compromised individuals. Village ponds are also crowded with cattle and rank vegetation and used indiscriminately for bathing, cooking and even for drinking water.

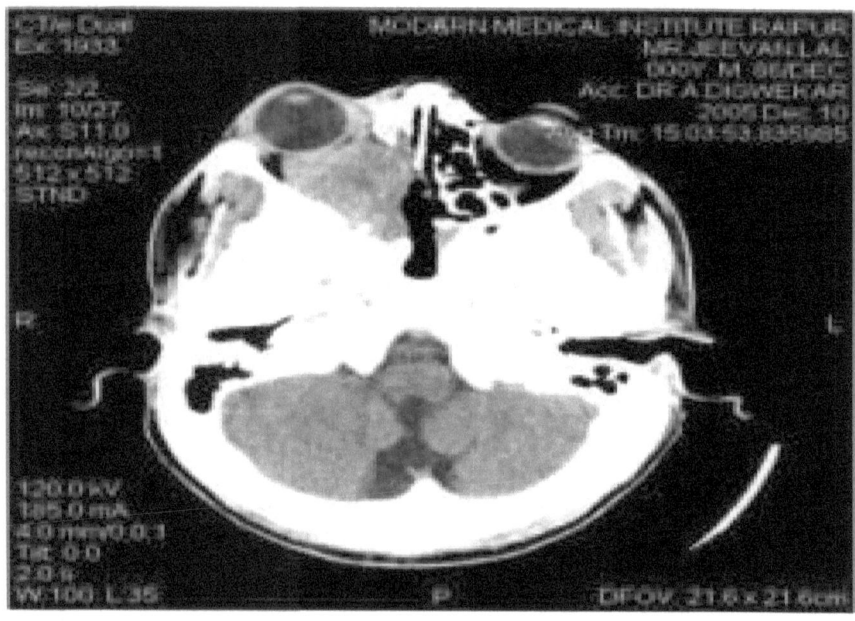

FIG 19: A fungal ball sitting behind the right eyeball has also invaded the nasal sinus space. JLB, who came from the village of Palari, was diagnosed with orbital and nasal fungus *aspergilloma*. He was operated on in August 2005 and started on anti-fungal medication and amphotericin. But the same was stopped, as he developed jaundice. In December, he started experiencing headaches, lethargy and subsequent coma, leading to his readmission. A CT scan performed on admission showed a fungal

ball behind his right eye, involving the space behind the nose and invading the brain. He was treated with a newer drug called *voriconazole*. The initial week of intravenous medication was followed by a course of oral capsules. Fortunately, he showed considerable improvement. The brain compartment cleared of fungus; however, the orbital mass persisted. He was asked to continue with the oral medication, but then, he faced financial hardship and had to sell off his farmland. The approximate cost of the drug per month was over 50,000 Indian rupees (around 1000 US dollars), well beyond his means.

NOTES

1. *'The king's headscarf is the washer man's loin-cloth.'*

2. *"A person enjoying the position of first violinist in a string band which performs at Parsi weddings and on other festive occasions cannot evade the necessity for [a] clean shirt. The demand was fulfilled by [the] Dhobi who finds a shirt of the best quality for an evening in much less cost compared to [a] new one."*

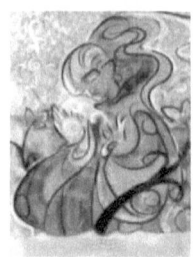

10 Stiff Spine & Tetanus

The soil in tropical countries and in India in particular is known to be much more infected with tetanus than in the case in temperate climates.
[The office of the Public Vaccinator, Correspondence; BMJ; February 1907]

Tetanus is an infection of the nervous system caused by the potentially deadly bacteria *Clostridium tetani* (*C. tetani*). Spores of the bacteria live in the soil and are found worldwide. In spore form, *C. tetani* may remain inactive in the soil, but can remain infectious for more than 40 years.

Contamination of deep, penetrating wounds was common in non-vaccinated warriors during times of war. The British Army adopted the practice of passive immunisation of wounded soldiers. This served the military well in the war of 1914–18, before the policy of active immunization came into practice. The large forces from Great Britain, India and New Zealand, were highly immunised in the 1940s, and the incidence of tetanus was only 0.13 per 1000 injured soldiers.

Tetanus infections were also contracted in operation theatres due to imperfect sterilisation. Tetanus was a much-dreaded sequel to caesarean sections, which were performed if complications developed during normal labour. Neonatal tetanus was yet another problem which resulted from the cutting of the umbilical cord with a rusted razor blade, after a home delivery. The death rate for newborns with untreated tetanus was even higher. Injuries caused by rusty nails were a common cause of tetanus among the barefoot population.

The time between infection and the first sign of symptoms is typically one to three weeks. Without treatment, one of four infected people die. But with proper treatment, less than 10% of infected patients die.

Some eminent veterinary surgeons in Calcutta used hemp resin in five cases of horses suffering from tetanus. Of these, three recovered. Another doctor cured a pony in a similar way. W.B. O'Shaughnessy, submitted clinical details to the Western world, of the treatment given to several patients afflicted with hydrophobia, tetanus and other convulsive disorders, in which a preparation of hemp was employed with good results.

CASE-1
The second case was that of Chunoo Syce (treated by Mr O'Brien, at the Native Hospital), in whom tetanus supervened on the 11th of December, after an injury from the kick of a horse. After an ineffectual trial of turpentine and castor oil in large doses, two-grain doses of hemp resin were given on the 26th of November. He consumed in all 134 grains of the hemp resin and left the hospital cured on the 28th of December. [O'Shaughnessy, W.B. *On the preparations of the Indian hemp, or gunjah,* 1843]

CASE-2
Such prefatory remarks I am led to make, from having lately observed in the Lancet, of the 14th of December, 1844, an excellent report of a case of tetanus, terminating fatally, at Guy's Hospital... I should have advised, after deciding upon the treatment, the use of the extract (of the Indian hemp) in much larger doses at very commencement than we gave... [Inglis, J. *Case of traumatic tetanus – Exhibition of the extract of Indian hemp (cannabis indica) – Death – Autopsy; The Provincial Medical and Surgical Journal;* 1845]

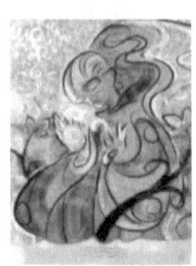

11 HEAT, DUST & MENINGITIS

May 31, 1829: How I rejoice this month is over; this vile month. It appears almost wicked to abuse the merry merry month of May, so delightful at home, but so hot in India. Mr M started from Calcutta... and died in his palkee of brain fever only three days afterwards, in consequence of the intense heat. [Parkes, F. *Wanderings of pilgrim in search of the picturesque; Residence at Cawnpore*; 1850]

The void created in many countries following the banning of the slave trade, was to some extent filled by the supply of untrained labour, mainly from India and China. These labourers created the Indian pockets in Guyana and Trinidad, the Indian Ocean islands and the Pacific. Outbreaks of meningitis occurred regularly at the port of Calcutta, where large numbers of labourers gathered prior to embarkation for the West Indies. The disease was also discovered in emigrant ships trading with the West Indies. Carter reported the first case of *pyogenic meningitis* in 1878 in Bombay and it was soon recognised all over India. During the first six months of 1934, 1991 cases and 1216 deaths were recorded.

Inmates of Indian jails were also periodically attacked with meningitis. Dimmock reported on the disease among the convicts of Shikarpur Jail during 1883–1884. In Chhattisgarh, a patient who was admitted at the Bilaspur Jail hospital in December 1927, died in February 1928. Major Buchanan worked in the central prison of Bhagalpur between 1897 and 1900 and recorded 47 cases over four years; of these, 32 patients died and only 15 fortunate inmates recovered. He also noted the presence of skin eruptions from herpes infection. The rashes appeared on the face or other parts of the body at variable periods during the illness but he attached no significance to it. Most of the cases occurred during the spring (March, April and May). He firmly believed that the germs were disseminated through dust in the spring or dry-weather months – especially in April, when dry, hot storms occurred daily, and winds blew steadily from 11am until 4pm. In fact, most patients worked at blue-collar jobs in dusty surroundings. Dust invaded everything and everybody in the summer and served as a vehicle for the germs that clung to old mats, walls and roofs.

The incidence of *cerebrospinal meningitis* gradually reached a peak at the beginning of the hot season. There was also a definite tendency for epidemics to die out with the increasing day temperatures. Regarding the decline of *cerebral meningitis* during late summer months, Russell noted: *The fact that many people sleep out of doors as soon as hot weather temperatures prevail may have some influence in causing the decreased incidence.* [Russell, A.J.H. *Cerebrospinal meningitis in India: The Indian Medical Journal*, 1936]

Today, outbreaks of mysterious viruses periodically cause *meningo-encephalitic* illness. There has also been an alarming rise in mumps cases in young adults who have not received the MMR vaccine. Mumps is a common cause of *aseptic meningitis*, with increased incidence in the spring.

Dr Sanders read an interesting paper before the Calcutta Medical Society in 1886, which recalled a case of fever with great hyperesthesia, swollen joints and *suppurative parotitis* diagnosed as *cerebrospinal* fever: *A special committee of Dr. C Leghorn as president and Drs Joubert and Clarke as members was appointed to investigate the matter, and we believe that the results of the enquiries and deliberations of this committee was a decided opinion that the disease in question was cerebrospinal fever or as it is also called epidemic cerebrospinal meningitis. Sixty-two cases were admitted into the hospital during the cold season, of which twenty-three died.* [Sanders. *Cerebrospinal Fever; Indian Medical Gazette;* May 1886]

ENCEPHALITIS LETHARGICA (VON ECONOMO DISEASE)
An epidemic occurred suddenly and extensively in Belfast in 1924 spring and early summer. The outbreak began in March; few cases at first, a large increase in mid-April, and continued till the end of June, when the epidemic ceased even more suddenly than it began. The total number of cases admitted during this recent outbreak was 183. The death rate in the last epidemic was 11.4 per cent. [Robb, A.G. *Encephalitis lethargica;* medical press and circular, *Indian Medical Gazette,* 4 March 1925]

Von Economo encephalitis spread across the world between 1915 and 1926. The disease left many speechless and motionless. Cases resembling *epidemic encephalitis* were first reported in India by the military medical authorities in Karachi as early as 1919. In response to such reports, the Director Medical Services in India issued a circular (dated 27 February 1920), to all Military Medical Officers in India, giving a brief description of the disease, with a view to enabling them to detect and treat cases as early as possible. The spread of epidemics in Europe created further panic among the authorities in India.

On 4 March 1925, Alex Gardner Robb described the features of the Belfast epidemics and published another circular in IMG: *In this epidemic, the prominent symptoms at the outset were as follows:*

(1) fleeting neuralgic pains; (2) nocturnal insomnia; and (3) mental excitement, restlessness and talkativeness. A little later, they developed the following: (4) double vision and other eye symptoms; (5) muscular twitching; (6) delirium of varying degrees; and (7) lethargy.

Herpes occurred in 6% of cases. Rapid and short breath and increased frequency of urination were also common symptoms. Dr Robb described himself as very sceptical about the quoted recovery rate of 20%. He estimated 5% as being nearer the mark.

Reports of the development of Parkinson-like features after febrile illness, appeared in IMG even before the epidemic struck Europe (in fact, as early as 1904). In 1929, Dhunjihoy, then Superintendent of Ranchi Indian Mental Hospital, reported a number of cases of what was suspected to be *encephalitis lethargic*, in IMG. Cases differed markedly in their presentation. Most had predominant psychiatric features but some had Parkinson-like features. The disease commonly began with a febrile illness and in its milder forms, it was often mistaken for malaria, even when malarial parasites were not found on blood smear examinations.

CASE-1 (IMG-1904)
Sepoy Kaka Singh (a young Sikh, 22 years of age), of the Burma Military Police, was admitted to Myinmu Hospital, suffering from malarial fever of a severe remittent type. He stated that he had had a fever about 14 days before admission. A fortnight after admission into hospital, his fever declined, leaving him weak, anaemic and complaining of trembling in his extremities and difficulty in doing things for himself. On rising, all movements were slow and deliberate: head and chest bent forward, arms held apart from the sides and flexed at the elbows. Legs wide apart, his steps were short, producing hurried 'propulsion'. No malarial parasites were found in the blood. He had a long course of quinine… There seems to exist a doubt that this disease is caused by malaria, but in this case, it undoubtedly was. [Good, J. *A case of Paralysis Agitans, "Parkinson's Palsy" with a note on its causation*; February 1904]

CASE-2 (IMG-1935)
K (a single male, aged 25 years), was admitted on 17 October 1934, to King George's Hospital for the following: (1) weakness and rigidity in both lower limbs and an inability to walk; (2) a similar condition in both arms and in the head and neck; (3) drowsiness by day and insomnia by night for the past three months; and (4)

increased salivation for two weeks.

About three months ago, he became febrile, which lasted for a few hours and was accompanied by slight shivering. The following day, he had a second attack of fever for a longer period. This intermittent type of fever continued for ten days. He lost his appetite, lost sleep and became constipated.

His shoulders were round and bent forwards, and so was his body. The fingers were partially flexed at the *meta-carpo-phalangeal* and at the *inter-phalangeal* joints. The thumb was adducted and flexed over the index finger, as in paralysis agitans, except that thumb and finger tremors were absent . . . The blood report was negative for malarial parasites, yet since the clinical diagnosis of malaria had been established, the fever was controlled with quinine, atebrin and plasmochin. [Stott, H. *The use of Stramonium for the rigidity and drowsiness following encephalitis lethargica*; November 1935]

Dr Ghosh reported another case to BMJ in 1935. In October 1934, a young man aged 23 years, who had recently returned to England from India, had an attack of fever with headache and giddiness, for which he was hospitalised for three weeks. This fever was diagnosed as *cerebral malaria* with a positive blood film for the parasite. He never fully recovered from the effects of the fever, and was finally discharged and sent home. When evaluated later, in April of 1935, he displayed a rigid gait and slow, monotonous speech. He had the typical Parkinsonian mask. His brother noted evidence of *oculogyric* crisis; he described an episode in which his brother's eyeballs rolled back while watching a movie and persisted in that state till the next morning.

Post-encephalitis lethargica cases are reported in India, even in persons who have never travelled out of the country. Fortunately, the disease has remained sporadic in India and has never reached epidemic proportions.

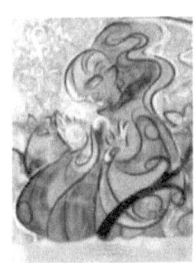

12 THE ANGRY GODDESS: SKIN SPOTS

Chronicle of a Calcutta epidemic:
July 17, 1824: A strong eruption came out, like the measles, and left me weak and thin. My husband's fever left him in thirty-six hours, but he has unable to quit the house for nine days; the rash was the same. Some faces were covered with spots like those on a leopard's skin. It was so prevalent, that the courts of justice, the Customhouse, the lottery office and almost every public department in Calcutta were closed in consequence of the sickness. In the course of three days, three different physicians attended me, one other having fallen ill. It is wonderful, that a fever producing so much pain in the head and limbs, leaving the patient weak, reduced and covered with a violent eruption, should have been so harmless; after three weeks, nobody appeared to have suffered, with the exception of two or three children, whom it attacked more violently than it did grown-up people, and carried [them] off.

Sept. 1st: The fever has quit Calcutta and travelled up the country state by state. It was amusing to see, upon your return to the course, the whole of the company stamped, like yourself, with the marks of the leech upon the temples. [Parkes, F. *Wanderings of pilgrim in search of the picturesque*]

Edward A. Jenner vaccinated a boy against smallpox in 1796. His work saved millions of lives. In earlier times, the practice of inoculation against smallpox was widespread across Persia, China and India but they all adopted different methods of inoculation.

Inoculation has been practiced in China since the time of the Tung Dynasty, and it was carried across the plateau of Central Asia to Turkey by herds of nomadic Tartars about 1000 years ago. Not more than 1% died of the inoculated disease. The inoculations were accompanied by strict dietary restrictions. The smell of whiskey, opium, heated *kang*s, and dirty or decaying matter, were to be religiously eschewed. For at least 100 days after inoculation, certain kinds of fish, eggs, beans and bean flowers, were avoided. Three years after the inoculation vaccination, buckwheat and cherries were to be shunned. Mr Pearson, a surgeon, introduced vaccination in China in 1805, although the Russians around Peking practiced it on a small scale before that. Vaccination was not favoured in Persia and inoculation, or the direct communication of the disease, was effected by placing the patient in the same bed with one suffering from small-pox of the most virulent type.

Indians have been long aware of the fact that an attack of smallpox provided almost lifelong immunity. In Bengal and Orissa, pus was collected from the blisters of smallpox patients and stored for use the following year. The operation was preceded by a ceremony performed in honour of Mother *Sitala*. The patient was inoculated with the crust of smallpox on the right forearm of a male or the left forearm of a female. He/she was then confined for 21 days, after which, a mixture of turmeric, *neem* leaves and coconut oil, was rubbed over the body. The inoculated person (if he/she survived), developed immunity against smallpox.

Another method was to precipitate mild abortive attacks of smallpox by blowing dried crust of the smallpox lesion from a survivor, into the nostrils of the recipient. This was done with the help of a silver tube placed in the right nostril if the recipient was male and the left nostril if the recipient was female. The procedure resulted in a mild attack of smallpox (if at all) and subsequently provided prolonged immunity to the recipient. Indeed, it was a tough challenge to replace inoculations with effective vaccinations until inoculations were prohibited throughout the country.

Mother *Sitala* is associated with certain epidemic diseases like smallpox. Her protection is called for when a village is attacked by an epidemic. The name she is called by depends on the size of the eruption: *Badi Mata* (large eruptions/smallpox), *ChotiMata* (small eruptions/chicken pox) or *Sendri Mata* (red eruptions/measles).

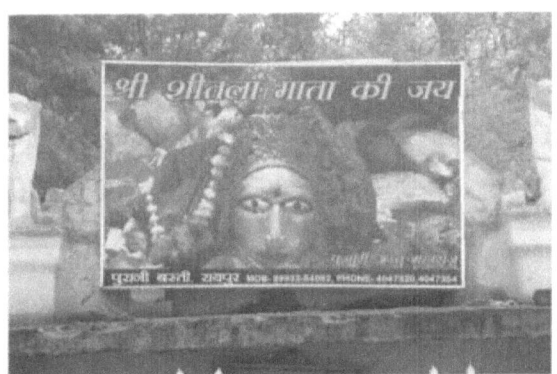

FIG 20: Goddess *Sitala* temple, Raipur. In Sanskrit, the name *Sitala* means 'the cold one'. She is primarily worshipped in the dry seasons of winter and spring, which is also the time for smallpox. This statue of Mother *Sitala* is made of silver and weighs about 12 *tolas* (one *tola* = ½ ounce).

Spring brings with it chicken pox (*varicella*), the disease caused by *varicella zoster virus* (VZV), along with its related complications. *Varicella* is one of the classic diseases of childhood, with the highest prevalence being in the age group of four to ten-year-olds. But in rural India, *varicella* is predominantly an adult disease. VZV can also lead to multiple other neurologic and ocular disorders. Sub-acute *Sclerosing Panencephalitis* (SSPE), a delayed complication of the reactivation of the measles virus, presents a changing pattern. More and more patients in the adult age group are being diagnosed with SSPE, and most of them were not vaccinated in childhood (in Chhattisgarh, those who were vaccinated, constituted about 40%). The effective vaccination of millions of children in a diverse geography, is a challenging task.

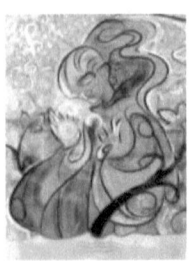

13 Dogbite & Rabies

Rabies is an infection of the central nervous system caused by *lyssavirus*, of the *rhabdoviridae* family. The virus is usually transmitted through dog bite and produces one of the most fatal viral encephalitides. At least 40,000 deaths are reported annually.

Apparently, the reason for the relatively higher incidence of rabies is the high number of stray dogs in India. These dogs form gangs and distribute their territories in towns, rather like the *mafiosi*. The stray dogs usually bark and run to bite on being disturbed by movements, usually late at night, during the breeding season. A slight seasonal rise in the prevalence of human rabies in India has been noticed during the monsoon. A dog's behaviour changes quite rapidly (usually within 10 days), under the influence of the bullet-shaped *rhabdovirus*. A vigilant dog becomes dumb and prefers isolation, his bark becomes either mellow or quite furious and he runs toward his own death and bites everyone in his way—whether cattle or human. The development of rabies in humans leads to certain death.

One of the earlier methods for dogbite, was the practice of excision of the *cicatrix* (wound clearance), in the belief that it would clear the remaining rabies virus, rather like snake poison. People still prefer crude *cicatrix* burning and cutting along with the application of indigenous herbs, in order to avoid the treatment with 14 injections in the anterior abdominal wall, using an older vaccine widely popular in India in earlier times.

In 1893, a project was planned to open a Pasteur Institute in India, so that people bitten by rabid or suspected rabid dogs, did not have to make the long journey to Paris. In July-August 1900, the Indian Pasteur Institute for the treatment of rabies opened in Kasauli. Lieutenant Colonel Sir David Sample, the then Director of the Central Research Institute, Kasauli, described an inactivated carbolised rabies vaccine that was used to treat over 2000 Europeans in India with a failure rate of only 0.19 %. The vaccine was called the Sample Vaccine. The vaccine was a remarkable success story even in its first year; 321 patients were relieved of their symptoms, and there were only three fatalities. The number of patients treated slowly increased to 543 in 1902 and 584 in 1903, with six deaths of severe (class-C) bites, where the nervous system had been affected before completion of the vaccination.

Kasauli became a popular place and people travelled from great distances for the rabies treatment. Indian patients were referred by letter with all details regarding the manner in which they had been bitten. The course of treatment ordinarily lasted 14 days and involved drug delivery by hypodermic syringes poked into the stomach wall. No patients were hospitalized for vaccination. They were housed at suitable hostels, boarding houses or lodges.

From 1912 to 1916, 22,519 people applied for the treatment at Kasauli. In 1916 alone, 5360 patients received the vaccination. Out of those who received treatment, 70 suffered from rabies, and the proportion of failures was only 0.8 %. However, the problem with the Sample Vaccine was and is, its allergy to animal neural protein, which causes *demyelination* in human nervous tissue. Almost one of every 10,000 cases is diagnosed with *allergic encephalomyelitis*. These complications have been reported on and off in medical literature since the 1930s. The following is an interesting case study.

On the sixth of April, 1932, a healthy-looking Anglo-Indian lady, aged thirty-one, came to see one of us (H.S.C.) with the following history: On about the 27th March, 1932, the sight of her right eye began to go dim, and three days later, her left eye began to go dim also. . . The left pupil was quite inactive to direct light, and there was no consensual reaction. The ophthalmoscope showed a typical **papilloedema** *of both discs. Apart from her very natural mental distress, she was not ill . . . She was put on mercury, potassium iodide and strychnine injections . . . Towards the end of the second week of her stay in hospital, she said the sight of her left eye was coming back . . . She was discharged at the end of two months with full vision (6/5) and full fields in her right eye. Her left eye was the same except that small* **centrocaecal scotoma.**

In the past:
The patient, a healthy and normal woman, was bitten by a dog, which was certified rabid, on March 3, 1932. She reported at the Pasteur Institute, Rangoon, on the fifth of March, two days after the injury . . . She was given class III treatment (i.e. 5 c.cm of a 5 per cent carbolised sheep vaccine) daily for fourteen days, receiving in all 3.5 grams killed sheep fixed virus. She attended regularly from the fifth of March for her treatment, which was completed on March 18, 1932.

The question as to whether this case is an example of the so-called 'post-inoculation paralysis' is a very interesting one. As is well known, antirabic inoculation is occasionally followed by disorders of the nervous system... In a personal communication to one of us, Lieutenant-Colonel H.E. Shortt, I.M.S., Director, Pasteur Institute of India, Kasauli, states that he recollected seeing a report in which optic neuritis had been observed in animals after antirabic treatment; but he, too, was unable to find the actual reference. [Cormack, H.S. Double Papilloedema Following Antirabic Inoculation: Recovery; Indian Medical Gazette; 1933]

At present, newer vaccines are being marketed at prohibitive cost. The treatment of rabies remains elusive. Various claims have been made for rabies cures by some of the most imaginative and exotic methods. Meanwhile, Ayurveda claimed to possess the ability to identify people who will eventually develop rabies after dogbite. Some bizarre methods of treating rabies by achieving hypersalivation, were also recorded. The following two atypical examples will illustrate the point.

CASE 1

The next morning, symptoms of hydrophobia completely set in. On admission, the paroxysms were very violent and frequent, the smallest noise or touch bringing on the spasmodic attack. I had him bound onto a cane-bottomed chair, surrounding him with blankets from the neck downwards, and I placed under the chair a large vessel of hot water; and one drachm of mercury, rubbed up with the same quantity of sulphur was also put under the chair in the piece of earthen chatee over a charcoal fire. Fifteen grains of calomel were given at once, and five grains repeated every hour afterwards. The mercurial vapour bath was kept up until all symptoms subsided. In about four hours, the patient was quite composed and free from all spasmodic symptoms, but was profusely salivated. [Barnes, J.J. *A case of hydrophobia successfully treated by salivation; Indian Medical Gazette*; 1868]

CASE 2

On the eighth of May, 1891, a middle-aged gentlemen, a well-known pleader of Meerut, while on a visit to his home at Jalandhar was bitten by a dog on his left leg . . . I excised the cicatrix on the eighth of June and kept the sore open for two weeks . . . On the seventh of August (i.e. fourteen weeks after being bitten), at 7 in the evening, while he was at a friend's house, he was suddenly seized with a violent spasm of the whole body, commencing from the left ankle, the spasm ran along the spine, passing to the face and the jaws . . . I saw him at 9 PM. The spasms were frequent and of a clonic character . . . At about 10:30 in the night, I got the pilocarpine solution ready, and injected 1/5 of a grain of the drug. The effect of the medicine was almost instantaneous—he felt warmer, was covered with perspiration, his mouth, dry so long got moist, and full of saliva, which he swallowed. The spasms, too, diminished greatly, and he felt much relief. [Ghose, N.T. *A case of hydrophobia cured by subcutaneous injection of hydrochlorate of pilocarpine; Indian Medical Gazette;* November 1891]

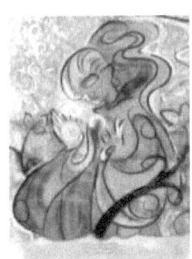

14 SNAKEBITE

The Indian Mongoose: He fought with the mighty cobra deep inside the Indian jungle and won the game. Soon afterwards, he consumed some herbs and rubbish for survival from the near lethal bite and venom of the deadly snake. On some other day, he was trapped by an Englishman, kept in a cage and bitten by a cobra in a controlled fashion for an experiment. No herbs were available as an antidote, and the poor Mongoose died.

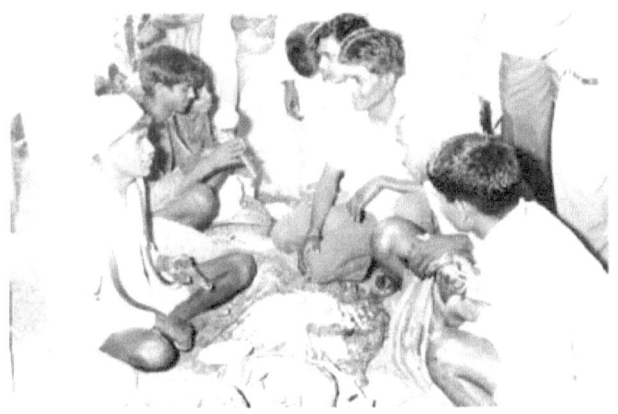

FIG 21: Snake charmer at a *Hindu festival.*

A LAND OF SNAKES

The British in India lived in perpetual fear of snakes emerging from every corner of the house, gardens, verandas, toilets, kitchen-shelves, and even beds. Snakes did have the most disconcerting tendency to emerge, slithering on the roads during an Englishman's morning walk, or accompanying him on rides in the coach. A story by Rudyard Kipling featured a Mongoose that saved an English family from two deadly cobras. The Indian Mongoose became a popular pet for protection.

Scientists conducted and published the results of multiple experiments with snakebite. They judged the effect of poisonous snakebite on other snakes, fowl, the Indian Mongoose as well as dogs, in search of an antidote. In the late 19th century, the Government launched a drive to eliminate snakes by offering rewards to the catchers of venomous snakes. The number of snakes brought in for reward was so high that the initial prize of eight *annas* per piece was reduced to three *annas*. Rewards continued to be offered in many districts, but the amount offered was as small as the cost of one pie (equal to half a farthing), for the killing of a venomous snake (**Appendix-5**).

ENGLISH REMEDY

Mr Hood, writing on the subject of snakebite in the *Lancet* in 1868, said that no antidote was required and all that was necessary was continued and forced exertion. He suggested: *So long as we maintain the action of the heart and lungs, the patient cannot die.* It is stated that Dr Spilsbury, former Physician General, Calcutta, tied a man who had been bitten by a snake, behind his buggy, making him run several miles.

The other way out was to keep the person awake with sustained stimulation until the effect of the venom disappeared. As noted by Mookerjee in the *Indian Medical Gazette* in 1968: *The treatment consisted of inhalation of a mixture composed of ammonia every ten minutes and the continual pouring of cold water over the head. In the course of an hour, she became conscious, and her pulse seemed improved. She was then ordered to be continually shaken and loudly spoken to in order to remove the lethargic state from which she was still suffering, and at the end of a couple of hours from her admission, she was perfectly cured.*

SNAKE STONE & TANJORE PILL

On the other hand, natives attained similar success in treating snakebite with their own empirical methods. One of these involved the use of small pebbles with the capacity to draw out the poison from the wound, as well as various herbal decoctions.

In this town of Diu the so much famed Stones of Cobra are made; they are composed of the Ashes of burnt roots, mingled with a kind of Earth they have and once again burnt with that Earth, which afterwards is made up into a Paste, of which these Stones are formed. They are used against the stinging of serpents and other venomous Creatures, or when one is wounded with a Poisonous Weapon. A little Blood is to be let out of the Wound with the prick of a Needle, and the Stone applied thereto which must be left till it drops off of itself...

Scarification; suction of the wound; tight ligature and topical application of herbs on bitten areas; chewing leaves or barks; and drinking plant extract – all these formed the bases of ethnic treatment for venomous snakebite. In India, one of the mysterious methods of treating venomous bites was the application of a snakestone. These snakestones were usually small objects, jet-black, and made up of fragments of calcified bone, which, after calcination, were filled with blood and charred again. The upper surface was regular and slightly convex, while the lower was somewhat irregular and slightly concave; all the surfaces were highly polished. When applied to the punctured skin, it adhered to the surface. The power of snakestone lay in its ability to absorb venomous blood, due to its porous consistency and the fact that it consisted in part of animal charcoal.

The once-famous Tanjore Pill, contains a compound of white arsenic with black pepper and native herbs. It was considered an effective remedy and used officially in company hospitals of the Madras Residency. Patric Russell (1726–1805), 'Father of Indian Ophiology', also believed in the efficacy of the Tanjore Pill, and Mr Ireland treated five cases of poisonous snakebite with success.

The dramatic scene of treatment by indigenous methods was remembered for many years.

In the interval, a man had arrived on the scene, who at once assumed and was tacitly admitted by the bystanders to do so the treatment of the case. He quietly put aside the charmers, reassured the woman and her relatives with an air of perfect confidence as to the safety of her life, and pounding something on a stone, he administered it to her. We then left, directing that a report of the progress of the woman's case should be made from time to time . . . This case led me to make enquiries about the person who had treated it so successfully, and I sent for him. [Experiments on the action of snake poison and its antidote conducted at Gwalior Residency, in the presence of Colonel C.L. Showers, Officiating Political Agent, and Dr J. Macbeth, Superintending Staff Surgeon of Morar; *Indian Medical Gazette*; 1869]

SNAKEBITE IN CHHATTISGARH

The number of deaths due to snakebite in Chhattisgarh was estimated at 1,244 in 1911. Efforts were made to popularise the Lauder Brunton method to treat poisonous snakebite. The instrument was a small wooden lancet with removable caps at both ends and a central section to carry potassium permanganate crystals. The method involved rubbing the potassium permanganate crystals through the incised wound after ligation of the limb.

In this case, which occurred at (Durg), the victim, while in his hut at the village of Bhilai, was bitten in the toe by a snake. A basket was immediately placed over the reptile and information at once sent to the police station. A constable, who happened to possess a Lauder Brunton lancet, promptly proceeded to the hut and treated the puncture in the toe in accordance with the directions. Mr Crawford, Deputy Commissioner at Durg, saw both the man and the snake at the district headquarters on the following day, and the snake was clearly identified as a krait (Bungarus coeruleus).

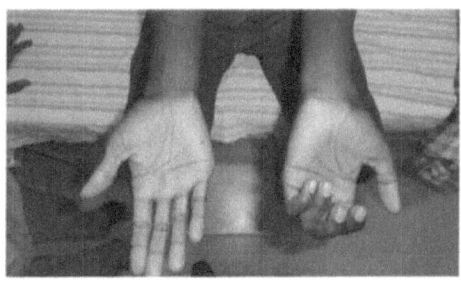

FIG 22: Left hand contracture resulting from tight ligature after snakebite. Hemant was bitten by an unknown snake while fishing at a local pond. There was a fang mark on his left palm at the upper transverse crease. He tied a tight band over his left arm for half an hour to prevent the spread of the poison. He developed a flexion deformity of the fingers due to the resultant lack of blood supply to the muscles. A moderately tight tourniquet application is required to prevent the spread of snake venom.

The largest population of snakes in Chhattisgarh state is found in the Farsabahar area of the Jashpur district, famously known locally as *Naglok* (Land of Snakes). The rainfall, vegetation and forests here suit snakes and it has become a breeding ground for many species of snakes. Over 10 people die from snakebite here every year. Novel strategies to repel snakes are utilised by those working in the fields, surrounded by venomous snakes. *Gumma bhaji* (Leucas aspera), commonly known as *dronpushpi,* is a common weed. It is generally believed in Chhattisgarh that if taken regularly, the body develops a specific smell which repels snakes. Villagers, particularly farmers, prefer this weed during the rainy season, when the incidence of snakebite is highest. Snakes gather around certain plants and the roots of these plants, called snakeroots, are traditionally used to cure snakebite, the principal drug being *Ophiorrhiza mungo*. The tribal population also uses the bark and stem of another snake-attracting plant called *brahmarmar.*

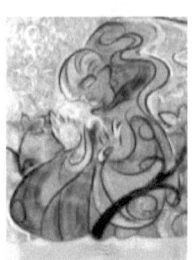

15 DEFORMITY

FRAGILE BONES

Others there are with their right arm brought round the neck over the left shoulder, and the left arm over the right shoulder, and their fingers clasping one another before their breasts, with the palms of their hands turned outwards. This twists the arms, dislocates the shoulder bones and therefore vexes the patient with inexpressible torments... [Ovington, J. The Faquirs near Surat: A Voyage to Surat; 1696]

Others with their arms dislocated so that the . . . joints inverted, and the head of the bone lies in the pit or valley of the arm... [Fryer, J. A Description of Surat: A New Account of East-India and Persia; 1698]

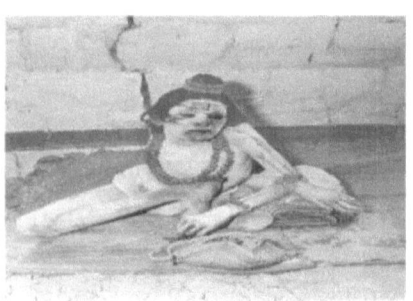

FIG 23: Odd posture with dislocated shoulder & hip joints, adopted by an individual with hypermobile joint at the *Kumbh Mela* 1965, Ujjain.

FIG 24: Odd posture with broken bones, adopted by an individual with *osteogenesis imperfecta,* at the *Kumbh Mela* 1965, Ujjain.

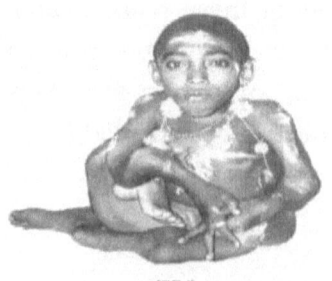

John Ovington set off from England on 11 April 1689, on board the ship *Benjamin*, and reached Bombay after 49 days, on 19 May 1689. John Frayer started on 9 December 1672, on a 12-month voyage from England, and reached Surat on board the ship *Falcon*, from Bombay. At the city of Surat, they both came across some saints and *fakirs* displaying distortions of limbs due to dislocation of joints, on the bank of the *Tapti* river. Contortion is the unusual skewedness of the human figure. It is achieved by an extreme degree of bending and flexion by contortionists. In some rare instances, they even dislocate the shoulder and hip joint to adopt a certain posture. Some of them have underlying defects in collagen or connective tissues that cause *ligamentous laxity*. The ability to stretch joints further than is normal is seen in medical conditions like *Ehler Danlos Syndrome, Hypermobile Joint, Marfan Syndrome* and *Osteogenesis Imperfecta*.

LEGEND OF ASHTAAVAKRA
At large Indian religious gatherings like the *Kumbh Mela*, many human oddities display their 'skill'. Some of them, with severe skeletal disorders, assume complex postures called *asana*s. Most of these people suffer from a rare collagen disorder. According to ancient Indian tradition, Ashtaavakra was an intelligent and spiritually advanced saint (whose wisdom has been a source of enlightenment through the centuries). He is believed to have existed in the 4th or 5th century BC and was cursed, while in the womb, with eight deformities. Thus, when he was born, he had eight bends in his joints, causing him to be named Ashtaavakra (Eight Bends). In modern medical parlance, congenital contractures of many joints, such as the ancient sage was afflicted with, is known as *arthrogryposis multiplex congenita*.

From ancient times, malformations in human beings and animals have attracted crowds. In ancient Egypt, deformity was viewed favourably, even as a mark of divine beneficence, thereby elevating those so affected from the usual social strata to important magico-ritualistic positions. Even acquired deformities were no barrier to holding high office in ancient Egypt. In contrast, the Greeks and Romans believed that deformed children were the expressions of curses or divine anger. The Romans used deformed slaves for entertainment. In fact, the demand for such slaves was so great that separate markets were set for their sale. In India, according to Dr Dinesh Mishra, older women, widows, and women with deformities or abnormal facial features, are often accused of being witches (*tonhi*) and barbarically persecuted in the villages of Chhattisgarh.

Even in the global scientific context, the malformed were referred to as 'monsters' in medical literature, until the early 1900s [1]. There has always been a common societal propensity to display human oddity as something wild and amazing – something from which the medical fraternity of yore was no exception. A procession of strange people from a circus were displayed in front of the medical community in January 1935 at Princess Beatrice Hospital, Kensington, London. There were the Giraffe-necked women from Penang; individuals with pituitary infantilism; the leopard-skinned women from Madagascar; and so on.

SMALL HEAD
At Shah Daulah's shrine in the city of Gujarat, Punjab, now in Pakistan, children and adults called 'rats' or 'mice', have existed for centuries. The shrine possessed the reputation of fulfilling the childbearing wish of barren women. Shah Daulah's 'mice' were curious types of imbeciles with micro-cephalic heads, which were sharply backward-shaped, producing a strange rat-like appearance. At an American circus, more than 20 micro-cephalic individuals performed as 'pinheads', popularly portrayed as 'missing links' or children from lost civilisations. It took time for a sense of public decency to prevail; and it was only in the mid-20th century that many American states prohibited public display and exhibition of people with mental retardation.

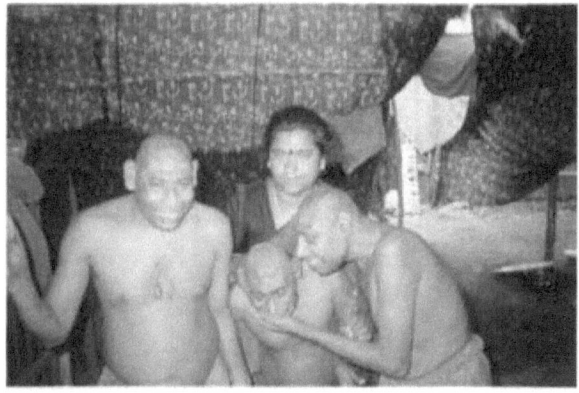

FIG 25: Ape gods. Three brothers with mental retardation and vertical folds on their heads (*cutis vertices gyrate*), at a fun fair.

Another Indian family case study is germane to the context. Three brothers with small heads and mental retardation, were displayed at a fun fair in a small city. They were deaf and dumb and imbeciles from birth, and they communicated through gestures. They resembled the fictional denizens of the *Planet of the Apes*, due to their short stature and the forward bend in their spines. Their scalps appeared in vertical folds as gyri appeared on the surface of the brain; hence the name of the disorder, *cutis vertices gyrate*, which is a term applied to the hypertrophy and parallel or gyrate folds of the skin of the scalp. The three brothers were dependent on caregivers for all activities of daily living. The eldest was about 51 years of age. The other two were in their 40s. The family hailed from south India. The other three brothers and two sisters in the family were normal. One of the normal siblings had adopted his three retarded brothers. They moved around the country with Mina Bazaar. During show time in the evenings, they would beat the drum and clap. Considering them to be monkey gods, the gathered crowd would offer them fruit and money.

One of the three was born with a small tail that was operated upon during his childhood. The human tail is another source of bewilderment in *Hindu* society. Children with such afflictions would disappear from follow-up as soon as they were scheduled for surgery, as any such intervention is held to be against the wish of the monkey god, Hanuman. Humans have tails that measure about one-sixth the size of the embryo itself. As the embryo develops, the growing body absorbs the tail. Infrequently, a child is born with a 'soft tail', which contains no vertebrae but only blood vessels, muscles and nerves. There have been few documented cases of tails containing cartilage, or even up to five vertebrae in length.

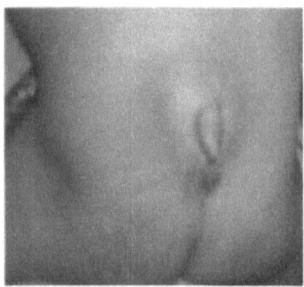

FIG 26: A tale of a tail. A male infant with a tail was scheduled for surgery but he disappeared from follow-up when relatives refused further treatment, considering such to be against the wishes of the monkey god, Hanuman.

Both the ancient Greeks and the Hindus believed in gods inspired by animal morphology. The Greek god Pan, is depicted with a tail emanating from his lumbar spinal area. Ancient Greek artists are quite accurate in their depictions of animal tails. The Pan tail is possibly based on an ancient observation of an abnormality associated with the lower spinal cord.

NOTE

1. Professors Jones and Eve of Nashville University have described an extraordinary monster, which is now living and, though infant, will likely reach maturity. It has four legs and two distinct female organs of generation, with two external openings of the urethra and two external openings of the double rectum. [An Extraordinary Human Monster; The Richmond and Louisville Medical Journal]

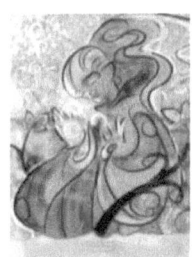

16 HYDROCELE TAPPING

LEAKY ION CHANNEL

My technique is to tap the hydrocele with an ordinary trocar and cannula as completely as possible and then inject 10 cubic centimetres of 1 per cent solution of quinine urea... Slight pain is experienced in the inguinal region for a minute or so, but nothing at all afterwards... The fluid is massaged all round, and then the patient is allowed to go home with instructions to report once a week. A second tapping is done... To beginners, I would suggest that the cannula should be driven well into the sac, as otherwise, there is the possibility of its slipping out into the cellular tissues during the manipulations of emptying it. [Vasavada, D.M. *Injection Treatment of Hydrocele. Indian Medical Gazette*; October 1931]

The practice of *hydrocele* tapping has existed since antiquity. This method involves the puncturing and draining of the *scrotal sac* for the palliative cure of the *hydrocele*; and at times, patients require repeated evacuation as soon as the sac fills up again. Recurrence is prevented by injections of various *sclerosing* agents into the *scrotal sac*. The instilling of chemicals results in adhesions and fibrosis inside the sac and eventually less collection of fluid. In 1903, Luke from Georgia, USA, cured several *hydrocele* patients and had with a high success rate using iodine and carbolic acid injections. Some surgeons injected 40 % alcohol, diluted in an equal quantity of water or a 10 % solution of zinc chloride, without the withdrawal of fluid. The procedures were frequently followed by recurrences. They injected all sorts of fluids, from milk to port wine, into the emptied sac. In the 1940s, *hydrocele* was treated by injection of *quinine urethane* by British surgeons. The usual complications included inflammation, haemorrhage and severe pain that persisted for a few days. The pain varied according to the chemicals used in the procedure.

Rural India is full of quacks who specialise in *scrotal hydrocele* tapping. They paste their posters of advertisement on public walls. But for the local villagers, it is a secret and relatively cheaper procedure when compared to surgery, which costs thousands of rupees.

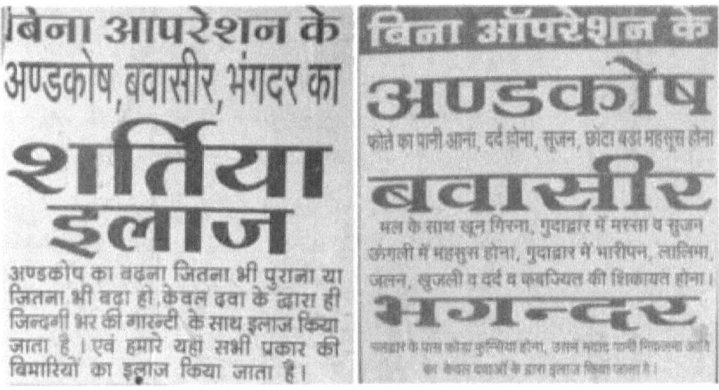

FIG 27: Public poster claiming cure for *hydrocele*, bleeding piles and rectal prolapsed, without operative intervention.

A male in his 30s, reluctantly gave the history of scrotal tapping by a quack for fluid collection during the months prior to reporting to us. It resulted in pain in the local area that subsided within a few days. Six weeks after the procedure, he was unable to sleep and became restless due to pain in the lower limbs. His thigh and leg muscles were rippling and moving in a wave-like fashion without reason. That, incidentally, was my first encounter with the syndrome. He recovered subsequently, and we were not able to correlate the *hydrocele* tapping and the subsequent involuntary movements.

Ten other cases have been recorded since 2003, of *hydrocele* tapping and the local instillation of drugs into the *scrotal sac* to prevent recurrence. The ages of the patients ranged between 28 and 47 years, and they had all undergone *hydrocele* tapping by quacks. The symptoms started 15 to 45 days after the procedure, with excruciating pain in the lower limbs, followed by a continuous rippling movement and gait disturbances. The condition of flickering muscles and restless behaviour is called *Morvan's fibrillary chorea*. These features were accompanied by marked anxiety, insomnia and visual hallucinations. They all had inflamed scrotums and they all recovered completely after a stormy course of the disease and sleepless nights.

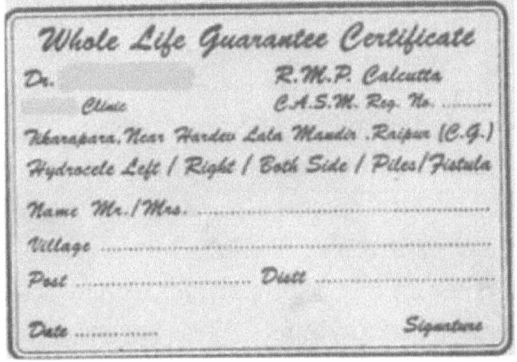

FIG 28: Guarantee card issued by a quack for assured *hydrocele* treatment.

Morvan's Syndrome is a rare autoimmune disease caused by the formation of antibodies against the voltage-gated potassium channel, named after the 19th century French physician, Augustin Marie Morvan. In 1890, Morvan described patients with multiple, irregular contractions of the muscles, cramps, weakness, excessive sweating, lack of sleep and restless behaviour. The syndrome is sometimes seen in association with tumours, and it exerts a remote effect. It is also believed to occur in cases of gold, mercury or manganese poisoning and after consuming indigenous medicines in India.

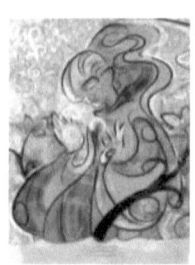

17 THE NERVE-TRAPPING INJECTION

May I again urge that the outer side of the thigh is the proper place for such injections? The vastus externus is a very large muscle; it is protected by the fascia lata and is not traversed by any important vessels or nerves. The muscular mass is of large capacity, and as much as 500 c. cm. can be introduced into its substance at a sitting provided the injection is made slowly and deliberately. [Turner, G.G. *The site for intramuscular injection*; BMJ; July 1944]

A four-year-old girl was evaluated in my clinic for weakness in her left foot. She was unable to walk and not even able to keep footwear on her left foot. She had reportedly received an injection in her buttock for a fever of two day's duration. She cried inconsolably and complained of tingling in her limb but her complaints had gone unheeded. She started limping the following day. The girl's mother, considering it the result of pain at the injection site, gave her hot fomentation, but the limping persisted. Finally, she was brought to the clinic. On examination, it was seen that a PIP (Post Injection Palsy) had resulted because of damage to the sciatic nerve. A large nerve had been damaged by a drug or needle beneath the layers of gluteus muscle.

In May 1988, the World Health Assembly asked for a commitment from member nations of the World Health Organization (WHO), to achieve the goal of global eradication of poliomyelitis. The *Acute Flaccid Paralysis* (AFP) surveillance programme was undertaken on a massive scale to identify all reservoirs that transmitted the wild polio virus. It included AFP case investigations and laboratory testing of stool specimens collected from AFP cases for the polio viruses, using specialised laboratories. WHO appointed a large and efficient taskforce of skilled personnel in India, who worked its way through the villages and conscientiously reported all incidents of sudden, floppy weakness of the limbs. The next step involved the collection of an adequate number of stool samples within two weeks of the onset of the paralysis for viral studies. Unfortunately, the late reporting of cases remained a major problem in the field.

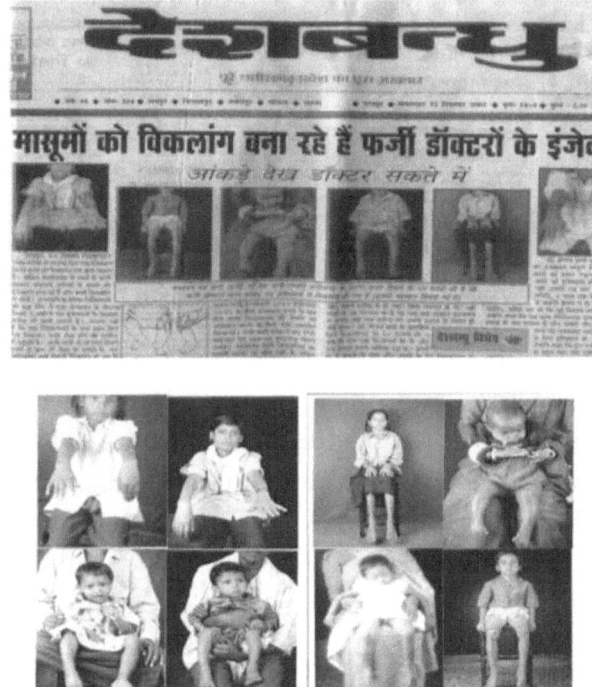

FIG 29: *Deshbandhu*, a popular daily newspaper, dated 31 Dec 2002, carried a cover story on post-injection palsy and wrist and foot drop, affecting a number of children.

The Nerve-Trapping Injection

In Chhattisgarh alone, 100 cases of limb paralysis were discovered in two consecutive years (2001 and 2002), due to faulty injection techniques. Of the 100 children, 40 were below the age of two years. Babies were traditionally received injections soon after birth and several times thereafter, to 'gain strength'. The injections were given deep in the buttock instead of being injected on the outer aspect of the thigh.

Administering medication through the intra-muscular route is a popular practice in rural India. A typical scenario consists of a child being held tightly by the in the mother while a needle and syringe is filled with a drug and poked deep into the buttocks. It is followed by a quick rub with a spirit swab, and it is all over. Parents are satisfied that this magical medicine via a shot will help cure fever and pain and/or give strength. Qualified doctors and quacks alike perform this procedure. Members of the rural society still perceive doctors as men with injections.

Intramuscular injection is one of the several methods used to deliver small amounts of medication. The drugs given through this route include antibiotics, analgesics, sedatives, anti- psychotics, hormones, vaccines and others. Depending on the chemical properties of the drug, the medication is absorbed in variable time and unpredictable fashion. Intramuscular injections are often given in the arm, buttocks or outer aspect of the thigh. In the case of the buttock, the injection site should be on the upper, outer quadrant to avoid damage to the large sciatic nerve.

Some drugs were more notorious than others, especially drugs that were not water-soluble. Cases were reported in which nerve lesions resulted from the injection of quinine near nerve trunks. After World War II, many soldiers were the victims of severe and persistent neuritis or paralysis affecting the great sciatic because of the injection of quinine solutions into the nerve instead of into the mass of gluteus muscle. In the 1940s, some practitioners strongly advocated the abandonment of the gluteal site for intramuscular injections and recommended the outer side of the thigh as the proper site for the procedure

Adhesions resulting from multiple intramuscular injections, at times trap a nerve in its vicinity. At least two kinds of nerve injuries have been noted: immediate palsy (with severe disabling pain at the time of penetration that possibly results from direct penetration of a nerve under the thin muscle mass of a child); and delayed palsy (which develops several days later, due to chemical injury and fibrosis around the nerve). Nearly 5 % of *acute flaccid paralysis* (AFP) cases are considered to be due to *post-injection palsy* (PIP). A follow-up of some such cases showed good recovery in the majority, while a few continued to limp – a rather high incidence of a completely preventable disability.

A study conducted in Hyderabad showed that 70 % of the injections prescribed were irrational or unnecessary and could have been substituted by oral drugs. Do children require intramuscular injections at all, apart from routine vaccinations?

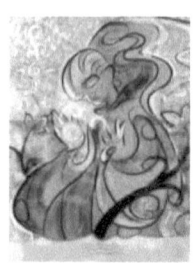

18 MEDICAL GEOLOGY: MANGANESE TOXICITY

Seventy per cent of Indian rivers are polluted. Underground water in 19 states is grossly contaminated. Air pollution in 90 per cent of Indian cities can cause respiratory diseases. Forests are depleting. We may survive the environmental hazards; our children will not. [State Environment Report India, 2009]

The new technological industries in the 1800s, required the following materials: oil, rubber and non-ferrous metals. By the end of the century, Russia, India and Chile were known producers of manganese. Central India is one of the world's richest manganese sources with underground and surface deposits. The inhalation of manganese dust leads to weakness, loss of appetite, irritability, lack of sleep and increased libido followed by mania, Parkinsonism and a kind of hilarious laughter called 'sham mirth'.

In February of 1956, the manager of a manganese mine situated in the district of Chhindwara, Madhya Pradesh, visited the office of the Regional Inspector of Mines, Chhindwara, and met Dr B.K. Sengupta, the then Junior Labour Inspector of Mines. The purpose of the visit was to determine whether he could dispense with the services of some of the underground workers employed in his mine, who, according to him, showed definite signs of mental imbalance and whose continued presence in the mine was unsafe both for themselves and their co-workers. He wanted to know if the Department of Mines could help him in such an action. It was suggested to him to send the patients to Nagpur Medical College Hospital or to the Civil Surgeon, Chhindwara, for diagnosis.

The manager, as advised, sent some of the patients to Nagpur Medical College Hospital, where they were admitted and kept for about a month under observation. The cases were diagnosed as *'shaking palsy'* and the patients were recommended 'rest'. When Dr T.P. Niyogi, the then-Civil Surgeon, Chhindwara, examined these patients, he suspected chronic manganese poisoning.

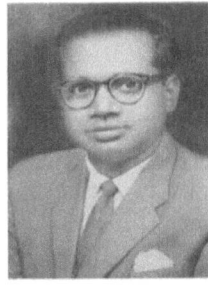

FIG 30: **Dr T.P. Niyogi** (22.03.1915 - 15.05.1991), did pioneering work on manganese toxicity among the miners of central India.

To corroborate the findings, a surprise inspection of the mine was conducted on 2 June 1956, and it was found that dry drilling was being done on the floor and sometimes also on the sides and roof of the mine. Three more cases were discovered amongst the drillers, who manifested similar symptoms. The manager was requested to send the new cases to Chhindwara Hospital for observation. After a period of close observation, Dr T.P. Niyogi diagnosed seven cases as chronic manganese poisoning – the first cases of manganese poisoning reported in India. One of them, it may be added, had been earlier diagnosed as insanity by a local physician and the patient kept for some time in Sausar Jail, Chhindwara district.

On 15 June 1956, the Junior Labour Inspector of Mines reported the matter to the Chief Inspector of Mines in India, through the Regional Inspector of Mines, Chhindwara. The Chief Inspector of Mines was requested to send Dr M.L. Rawal, Inspector of Mines (Medical), for a further detailed study of the cases in collaboration with the Chhindwara Hospital authorities. He visited Chhindwara on 13 July 1956, and examined some of the cases. He was also of the opinion that these were cases of manganese poisoning, and he submitted his report to the Chief Inspector of Mines in India, who in turn forwarded the report to the Ministry of Labour, with a request that a committee be appointed to investigate the matter. The Ministry agreed to the proposal and set up the Manganese Poisoning Enquiry Committee for Labour and Employment, Government of India [1]. The terms of reference of the Committee were as follows: *A complete investigation of causation, extent, diagnosis and treatment of the different varieties of manganese poisoning found in the workers of the manganese mines in India and to advise on the preventive measures that may be enforced.*

About 22 cases were encountered in 12 mines and 11 patients were further investigated under the guidance of Dr N.H. Wadia, at the Department of Neurology, JJ Hospital, Bombay. Some were treated and followed up, but no improvement was noted. More problems resulted due to water from sources that we normally consider safe for drinking. The groundwater rapidly became less and less in quantity and more and more contaminated with unwanted elements like fluoride and arsenic. Bone deformities due to 'fluorosis' are caused by drinking fluorinated water. The disease is confined to certain pockets in India. People from the state of Andhra Pradesh use tamarind to bind fluoride ions. This advantage, accruing from traditional eating habits was, however, lost following the modern use of tomato rather than tamarind.

NOTE

1. The following members constituted the Committee: Drs M.L. Rawal, M.N. Rao, N.H. Wadia, T.P. Niyogi, M.N. Gupta, M.K. Chakraborty and B.K. Sengupta.

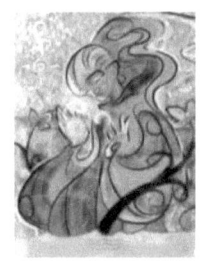

19 SUN, MOON & WEATHER

You may sleep out at night looking up to the moon till you fall asleep without a thought of moon blindness. [David Livingstone]

And straight the Sun was flecked with bars,	*One after one, by the star-dogged Moon,*
(Heaven's Mother send us grace!)	*Too quick for groan or sigh,*
As if through a dungeon-grate he peered	*Each turned his face with a ghastly pang,*
With broad and burning face.	*And cursed me with his eye.*

[Samuel Taylor Coleridge. Stanzas from *The Rime of the Ancient Mariner*]

A LUNAR OBSESSION
Long ago, the sun was nourished by the fresh water of the river, and the moon was fed by the sea. One day, evil forces captured the moon. They cooked their food on the moon and washed their utensils in the tides of the sea. The cooking and burning created toxic fumes on earth, which caused fevers. Even now, fevers fluctuate with the cycles of the moon, in coastal states, and dark spots caused by burning coal persist on the surface of the moon...

The extravagant stories narrated by writers of old, and the tales of sailors with regard to the influence of full moon beams, affected voyage psychology. Even though some did not consider these influences worth serious consideration, sailors (such as Coleridge's celebrated *Ancient Mariner*), believed in the existence of lunar power. Seamen who slept on the deck in bright moonlight, sometimes woke up in the morning with swollen faces. Other people, sleeping on the deck of a vessel, found themselves more or less paralysed when they attempted to rise. At other times, aches and pains occurred, resulting in an inability to move the limbs. It was later revealed that paralysis affected a person sleeping on the deck even when the moon was not visible at all. Instances of swollen faces were generally found to be related to *carious teeth*. Some varieties of ocular maladies – including complete blindness (*amblyopia*), night blindness (*nyctalopia*) or day blindness (*haemeralopia*), are presumed to be due to the strong lunar influence on sailors.

In the 1860s, there was the impression that malarial fever was aggravated by moonlight, especially in tropical climates. Based on their observations, Dr John Peet, in 1838, at the European General Hospital in Bombay, and Dr. Balfour in Bengal, emphasised that symptoms of intermittent fever occasionally worsened around the period of the principal lunar alterations, in coastal regions. Chatterjee published on the relation between lunar cycle alterations and elephantiasis, chronic rheumatism and chronic malarious intermittent fever. These observations led to further research by Moore and others, on periodic fevers, following careful observation of temperature charts in malaria-affected regions in the deserts of Rajasthan. No such association was noted in non-coastal regions by later researchers.

According to Lunarians, life, death, disease and even conception, all depend on the lunar cycle. Plague, asthma, hysteria, lunacy, epilepsy and haemorrhages, were all supposed to be under lunar influence. The association between phases of the moon and vascular diseases, arthritis and psychiatric disturbances, is still reported in current medical literature. A full moon reportedly produces agitation and outbursts of mania, unexplained stroke symptoms and exacerbation of gouty arthritis.

A day after the first solar eclipse of 2006, I was in discussion with a concerned father, whose ten-year-old son had suffered an epileptic fit the previous morning. I remember the father saying, with all the conviction of a true believer: *My son's sun sign is Scorpio, and this eclipse is considered particularly harmful for a person with a Scorpion sun sign, and so he had a fit.* The entire family had woken early (3 a.m.) on the day of the eclipse, to eat before the aura of the eclipse (*sutak*) started – a common practice among Hindus. The boy's father could not be convinced that the seizure was due to sleep deprivation. The family disappeared to seek cure/treatment at a shrine, even though the boy's CT-Head showed enhancing *solitary granuloma*, which looked like moons among the clouds. On another day, I remember a conversation with a drug-defaulter epileptic, who blamed the moon cycle for his seizures.

For many centuries, it was not possible to practice medicine without knowledge of astrology. In India, astrology continues to exist along with medicine. The stars govern the day and time of admission, surgery, and even discharge from hospital.

MORE PALPABLE EFFECTS OF SUN AND HEAT

May 20, 1866: He had fallen from his seat whilst at tea. The surgeon who was called to see him applied ice to the head and leeches to the nape of the neck and gave a powerful purgative, which took no effect. I saw the man almost directly after admission. He was speechless, his skin burning hot, pulse running, hardly to be counted. [Waller, W.K. Heat Apoplexy; Indian Medical Gazette; July 1869]

There has been more direct evidence of the influence of the sun and heat on human health. The post-mortem appearances of sunstroke patients show pathological changes in the scalp and subcutaneous tissues, as much as in the brain itself – all seeming to suggest that the victims had suffered from some sort of local 'cooking' of the head, with unpleasant results.

Early pictures depict the European soldier in a tight white overall and tighter red coatee, heavily braced with a belt, decorated with a lather stock, and the head covered with a forage cap with a calico cover and a poor sun flap behind – all of which was most uncomfortable and woefully non-protective in a hot climate. In contrast, the most characteristic feature of Indian apparel was the *pagri* (turban), the thick folds of which offer a significant protection against the sun for most of the head. These observations led to the introduction of the *sola topee* for protection against the sun and it replaced the impractical forage cap. The *sola topee* was a lightweight helmet made of pith from the *sola* plant (*Aeschynomene aspera*), and it was covered with cloth. The use of spine pads was based on the assumption that sunstroke was caused by the sun striking the spine. Initially, uncomfortable spine pads were designed but were gradually replaced by stylish, narrow strips of dark-coloured silk sewn inside the coat and provided a false sense of security to its wearer.

Between 1858 and 1867, over 1600 deaths were recorded due to apoplexy, and between1895 and 1900, around 4.8 % of deaths among European troops, were recorded as due to heat stroke, a disease that affected both those who were previously healthy and those with underlying fever, who were exposed to sun and heat. It is, of course, in the hottest months of the year that most cases occur and army statistics in India show that all *heat hyperpyrexia* occurs between May and September, with half the cases occurring in June. Male adults form the bulk of victims. In the army in India, British troops were more susceptible than the Indians, especially during the first two years of service; after that, there was another peak in the incidence curve at around 11 years of service. The high incidence during the first two years was due to lack of experience (of living in hot weather), and the second spike was due to increasing age, chronic disease and alcoholism.

The climate of Chhattisgarh is hot and humid due to its proximity to the Tropic of Cancer. It is completely dependent on the monsoon for rain. Summer in Chhattisgarh extends from April to June and can be uncomfortably hot, with the mercury hitting the high 40s. The hot atmosphere causes the onset of many diseases which are direct influenced by it. The summer season, with its high temperatures, brings many dramatic seasonal diseases to the region, like *periodic paralysis* and *cortical venous sinus thrombosis*.

A healthy young man became paralysed in the early hours of the morning. He had eaten plenty of rice with spices the previous night and was unable to move at all the next morning. The local doctor started him on a drip and referred him to a bigger hospital. Blood tests showed low levels of potassium. Correction of this imbalance resulted in a rapid recovery. The periodic paralysis problem resulted from a leaky ion channel in the cell. The disease is common in Chhattisgarh and attacks are often precipitated in the dry, summer season. It is characterised by paralysis of all four limbs; low potassium levels; raised muscle enzymes due to inflammation in the muscles; and an abnormal ECG. These cases are sporadic in nature, unlike the familial variety seen elsewhere in the world. The attacks are triggered by excessive daytime heat and sudden fall in the night temperature with lower humidity, and meals rich in carbohydrates (rice). For unknown reasons, cases of *sinus-venous thrombosis* are common on hot and humid days and mostly occurs in individuals with elevated homocysteine and low serum B12 levels.

In Ayurveda, paralysis is classified with arthritis (*rheumatism*). Sleeping in cold and damp surroundings was considered an important cause leading to *vascular catastrophe*. There were different drugs to treat paralysis caused by exposure to dampness and from paralysis in winter. Dr Forbes Watson, in a paper read before the Society of Arts in 1855, and printed in their journal, stated that during the course of a series of observations made in Bombay, India, on the direct influence of climate on the human body, he found that after a period of continued rain, as during the monsoon season, the blood deteriorated in a striking and remarkable manner, the chief alteration being found to occur in blood corpuscles.

Logg reported the following case in the *Indian Medical Gazette* in September of 1868: *The following case came under my observation during the winter of 1867: Miss O., a healthy, robust-looking girl, of florid complexion, with dark brown hair, aged fourteen, born and brought up in the hills, was attacked with hemiplegia of the right side of the body on the fifth of February, after exposure to a heavy rainstorm, while out for an airing the evening before...*

REMARKS BY THE AUTHOR: *As I have never seen or read of a case of paralysis occurring after cold and damp, I ask what the symptoms detailed above could be attributed to and which appear all the more remarkable for responding so readily to treatment.*

EDITOR'S COMMENTS: *We insert... what may be termed, the neat student's case. As our contributor's professional experience increases, he will doubtless meet many more instances of paralysis, as the result of cold and damp. We hope he will always have reason to be gratified with the same satisfactory results.*

NOTE

In regard to the impact of hot and humid conditions on humans, a new word, *hyther* was coined by W.F. Tyler. The word was used to indicate the joint effect of temperature and humidity upon human sensation. [*Hyther and Eugenics* IMG September 1904: 349]

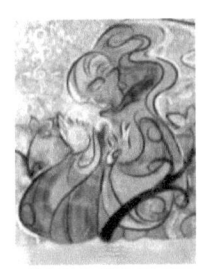

20 DESPERATE SYMPTOMS CALL FOR DESPERATE REMEDIES: HEADACHE

From loud talking and excessive talking, powerful scents, night-keeping, exposure to cold, physical exercise, suppression of the urgings of nature, fasting, violence done to the body, purging and vomiting in excess, from tears and grief and fear and alarm, from carrying of heavy loads and walking of long distances, the wind that is in the head increases and entering the veins of the head becomes excited. From the wind (thus excited) one gets a severe headache. [Sutherland, W.D. *Charaka Samhita*- Translated into English and Published by Avinash Chandra Kaviratna, Calcutta page 186; *Indian Medical Gazette*; February 1919]

Fanny Parkes, who lived in India between 1822 and 1846, is celebrated for her classic travel account. But, during her delightful journey, she was frequently troubled by migraine headaches. Many entries in her account, describe symptoms of this affliction and its exotic treatment modalities, including the efficacy of opium and piper betel leaf for headaches. Fanny Parkes also had, as a frequent accompaniment to her migraine, *mal de mer*, a French term for seasickness, which affected her on her sea voyage from Britain to the Indian subcontinent. She gradually learned about the environmental factors responsible for her headaches and about the Indian remedies to solve her problems. Day journeys under bright sunlight were perceived as a major precipitating factor. As noted by her on February 23, 1838: *The heat of the sun had given me a violent headache. I declined staying to see the King and requested permission to depart.*

An English gentleman observed that direct sunrays on the face resulted in the constant scrunching of the eyes and wrinkling of the brow to exclude the light. In one who did not wear darkened glasses, this was probably responsible for the majority of headaches. European men who sat hatless in tents on hot days, sometimes complained of headaches. Indian communities had different reasons for the precipitation of migraine attacks as compared to the Europeans. Exposure to cold (e.g. washing the head with cold water in the evenings), and missing morning tea (*chai*), often precipitated migraine attacks, more so among chronic sufferers.

In India, headaches have traditionally been treated using homemade remedies such as powder/paste of clove, cinnamon, garlic, ginger, almonds or henna flower extract, as well as application of sandalwood paste on the forehead; and consumption of betel leaf, cannabis and opium. Other remedies included washing hair with curd, massaging the scalp with medicated oil or *ghee* (preferably by trained hands), followed by adequate rest. Yoga has been found to be effective in cases of headache, and migraine symptoms have shown improvement with acupuncture. *Shirodhara*, a technique in which a pot filled with warm, medicated oil is hung over the head of the patient to allow a thick stream of oil to flow between the two eyebrows, is also known to effectively treat migraines. This is a popular procedure in Ayurvedic spas in south India and Sri Lanka.

Hypnotism and the practice of 'suggestion', probably had their origins in India, and were found to be quite effective in relieving migraines: *I have another patient who, for five years, suffered from daily paroxysmal unilateral headaches. Under treatment by suggestion (in the waking state), he has been free from headaches of any kind for the past eleven months, and he is apparently cured, all other previous treatments having failed.* [Nunan W. *Migraine and Suggestion; Indian Medical Gazette*, March 1928]

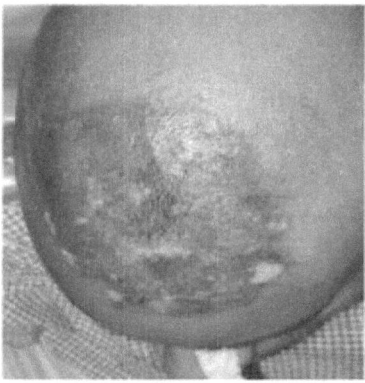 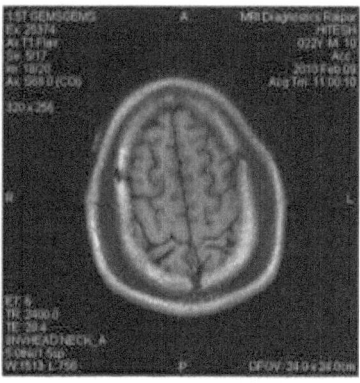

FIG 31: Large area of scalp burn and subcutaneous swelling detected on CT scan, resulting from application of hot clarified butter (*ghee*). A young boy was treated for his *meningitis*-related headaches with *ghee* on the scalp. This resulted in burns and the scalp tissue took days to heal.

After it was picked up from an Indian market, Indian hemp became a widely prescribed remedy for migraine and neuralgia in England and the United States from the 1880s to the early 20th century. At times it was mixed with *quinine hypobromide*, and sometimes with *scopolamine*, to treat neuralgia. After its discovery, even chloroform was used to calm patients who were in severe agony: *Some time ago, a lady, of about 45 years of age, consulted me about a violent headache, which every now and then attacked her and which she described as likely to drive her mad. From the lady's age, and other well-known symptoms, I unhesitatingly came to the conclusion that this very severe periodic headache was entirely due to the cessation of the menses. A few whiffs of chloroform from a pocket-handkerchief were recommended to be inhaled during the presence of a headache. Instant relief was afforded, and life was rendered bearable during the attack. Not only was the pain diminished and rendered bearable, but also the attack was shortened. From ten to sixteen drops of the anaesthetic were amply sufficient at a time . . . I have, on several occasions, and in a similar manner, administered these invaluable anaesthetics to patients suffering from severe headaches frequently accompanying intermittent fever. The relief afforded has been instantaneous and marked, and most agreeable to the patient.* [Elmslir, W.J. *Stray Notes on Chloroform*; January 1868]

Bayer, Germany, introduced *aspirin* in the Western market in 1899. The success of *aspirin* in treating migraine has effectively changed the story of treatment of headache forever, even in the most complicated cases of migraines.

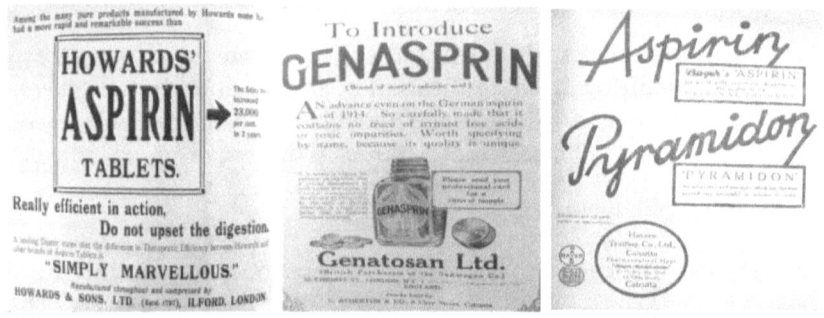

FIG 32: ASPIRIN was introduced by Bayer of Germany at the beginning of the 20th century. With the outbreak of World War I in 1914, the British market was immediately closed to German companies. Bayer faced stiff competition in all its major markets and multiple other brands were launched in India.

CHRONIC HEADACHE: A MODERN CASE STUDY

JLB records, at 66 years of age, his experiences with headache and the effect of aspirin: *It starts with a feeling of malaise for a while, say about 5 to 10 minutes. Thereafter, I see shreds of light swimming about in my field of vision. Then, my field of vision is strewn with dark patches. Consequently, if I have to read, 'I am going', I may see the line somewhat as, 'I m- ing'. Afterwards, I start losing my memory. In about 15 minutes to half an hour's time, I cannot recollect names, cannot tell time, cannot form words or sentences, cannot speak desired words nor can read, write or understand the spoken or written words. Speaking and thinking is possible sometimes with great mental effort only. Thereafter, half (the left side) of my body, including the tongue, becomes numb (similar to the condition that a limb may acquire on remaining under pressure for a long time).*

The condition described above remains for about 1 to 4 hours, after which, everything gradually returns to normal. The after effect of the attack is normally a feeling of weakness, constipation, headache etc. for about a week or two. A dull headache always remains.

The first debilitating attack came in 1953. At that time, I was under great tension due to domestic problems and problems from the employer's side. I was physically weak also due to poor nutrition. Ever since, I have suffered from the attacks off and on. There is no regular periodicity of the attacks. I am giving the dates of the last few attacks.

Angiography was done in 1957 at M.H. Lucknow. It did not show any pooling of dye or obstruction. A long time back, a doctor friend had advised 10 grains of aspirin as soon as the feeling commenced. The aspirin prevented the attack 9 out of 10 times. My mental agility and faculty is going down by each affliction. I have to exert double the mental strength to understand written or spoken words as well as to gather and channel my thoughts in day-to-day life. [Significantly, JLB's two subsequent magnetic resonance angiographies, done at the ages of 74 and 86 years, revealed no vascular malformation.]

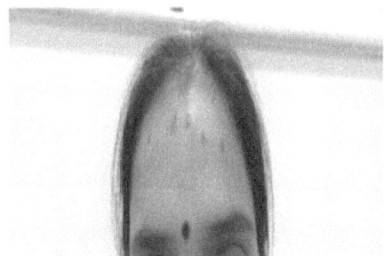 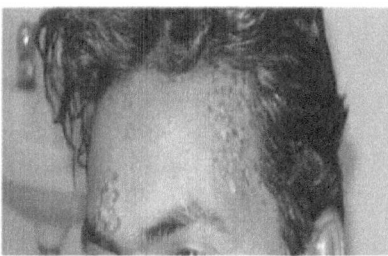

FIG 33: Pattern of burning & branding of forehead for migraine headache.

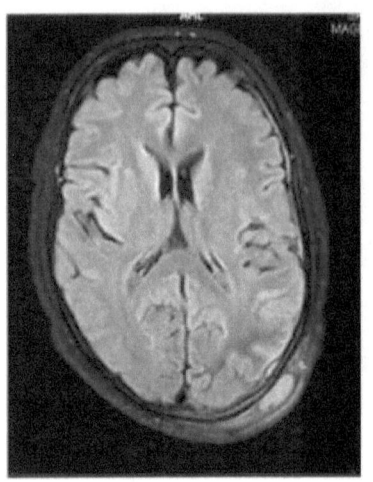

FIG 34: Barber's thump that fractured skull – blood collected underneath scalp and on surface of brain. A 36-year-old man undertook head massage and thumping by a barber, for relief from his headache. Unfortunately, the headache became more severe and localised to his left *occiput*. Examination showed local swelling and tenderness. An MRI of the head revealed a fractured left occipital bone. Collection of blood was noted under the scalp and on the surface of the brain.

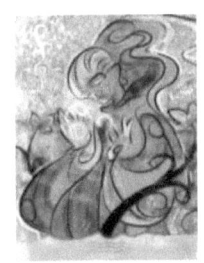

21 Epileptics in Lunatic Asylums & Drugs to Treat Epilepsy

It is an undoubted fact that epilepsy sometimes produces mental derangement of a furious kind. Because of its violent and destructive character, this is one of the most dangerous forms of insanity. The excitement or mania may last a few minutes, a few hours, or a few days; it then subsides, and the person coming to himself again appears as sane and rational as ever. [Firth, R.H. *Epileptic Insanity; Indian Medical Gazette*; April 1886]

During the first half of the 19th century, epilepsy was classified as a form of insanity. As a result, in lunatic asylums, there were some people confined among the insane, who suffered from epilepsy. The association of madness with epilepsy produced a rather negative image of epileptics. Multiple mental problems were identified in epileptics and thought to be dangerous to society. These included maniacal excitement, mental aberration and homicidal mania. The mental symptoms of epilepsy were grouped as follows:

1. Epileptic idiots: persons whose intellectual faculties have never been developed.

2. Epileptics who are imbeciles or demented: when paroxysms of epilepsy are very frequent and severe, and the disease is of a long duration, it generally impairs the intellectual faculties.

3. Epileptic maniacs: during the intervals between epileptic paroxysms, they are subject to fits of a manic nature.

The Medical and Sanitary Department during British rule, established lunatic asylums across the Indian subcontinent. The first asylum was opened in Calcutta prior to 1707, and then another opened in Madras in 1794. The Agra Asylum came into existence in 1859, which was renamed the Agra Mental Hospital in 1925. The British established an asylum at Ranchi on 17 May 1918 and named it Ranchi European Lunatic Asylum. It became the premier centre for mental health in the country and drew most of central India's psychiatric patients for treatment. These asylums provided in-door facilities for both criminal and non-criminal lunatics. In the 1901 census, 66,000 Indian people were noted as insane, out of a population of 294 million (0.02 %). In the five-year span ending 1900, the average lunatic asylum population was only 4,600. The low incidence of insanity among Indians was attributed to the lower prevalence of alcoholism, the lack of aberration due to religious terror and *'the fact that they possessed less brain energy than the inhabitants of modern Europe'*.

The statistics from lunatic asylums, as entered in the *Imperial Gazetteer*, reveal the percentage of epilepsy among lunatics at some of the asylums. This data does not include all the lunatic asylums in India. At times, the data was combined with other illnesses and so prohibited definitive conclusions. Also, the records of alleged causes of insanity were sometimes written by the police and had little scientific value. Nevertheless, they provided some insight into the problem of epileptics in the society of the time (**Appendix-6**).

There were four lunatic asylums in the United Province –at Bareilly, Lucknow, Agra and Benares – with 1148 inmates in 1903, of which 281 were criminal lunatics. Of the 327 cases in 1903, the principal causes of insanity were alleged to be *charas* and *ganja*-smoking (51); spirit-drinking (13); fever (28); epilepsy (23); heredity (17); exposure and injury to the brain (14); moral causes (46); and unknown (108).

In Lahore, the daily average number of inmates in 1904 was 554. Of these cases treated in 1904, in which a cause could be assigned, 16.59 % were attributed to the excessive use of Indian hemp in one form or another; 8.09 to epilepsy; 0.71 to heat; and 7.09 to mental causes, such as grief, worry and disappointment.

The Central Province, including Chhattisgarh, had two lunatic asylums, at Nagpur and Jabalpur, both of which were opened in 1866. In 1904, they contained 290 lunatics. Of the 306 cases in whom insanity was traced to a definite cause, 29 were shown as hereditary, congenital or due to a secret vice; 17 as occasioned by epilepsy or sunstroke; 30 by the consumption of drugs and spirits; 13 by fever; and 55 by mental distress.

In Assam, during the decade ending 1901, there were 350 admissions. In 232 cases, the cause of insanity was unknown; in 45 cases, *ganja* was said to be the predisposing cause; in 16, epilepsy; in 12, fever; in 10, spirit drinking; in 2, heredity; and in 9, opium.

In Madras, of the 769 cases admitted during the five years ending 1902, the history of only about half the cases was ascertainable. Of this number, exactly half had become insane from fever, epilepsy or other physical causes (25%); opium eating was the cause of five of the 769 cases.

[Extracts from the *Imperial Gazetteer of India Report* (1901–1904)]

The percentage of epileptics in asylums remained between 4.57 and 8.09%. The prevalence of psychosis in the general population ranged between 1 and 2 %The prevalence of psychosis between seizure attacks in non-selected epilepsy population studies, varies from 3.1 % to 9 % in current literature, and somewhat matches the earlier records of the asylums. This data from the asylums in the late 1800s and early 1900s, reflects the magnitude and difficulty involved in managing epileptics in society before the advent of effective medication to control seizures.

The search for a drug to sedate psychotic patients resulted in the discovery of some of the earlier antiepileptic drugs. Convulsions were successfully controlled by cannabis, and the use of *cannabis indica* was advocated in England, for its lighter sedative and tranquilising properties. It was conceptualised later to combine Indian hemp with bromide, to treat epilepsy, as this lessened *bromism* due to its diuretic effects. The idea was to use the combination, both in cases of chronic mania and epilepsy. Sedative, tranquilizer and poison[1,] all became potential anti-epileptic medicine.

...a single drop of the spirituous tincture, equal to the one-twentieth part of a grain in weight, was placed on the child's tongue at 10 PM. No immediate effect was perceptible, and in an hour and a half, two drops more were given. The infant fell asleep in a few minutes and slept soundly till 4 PM, when she awoke, screamed for food, took the breast freely and fell asleep again. At 9 AM, on the first of October, I found the child fast asleep, but easily roused – the pulse, countenance and skin perfectly natural. In this drowsy state, she continued for four days, totally free from convulsive symptoms in any form. During this time, the bowels were frequently spontaneously relieved, and the appetite returned to the natural degree... The child is now (December 17) in the enjoyment of robust health and has regained her natural, plump and happy appearance. [O'Shaughnessy, W.B. *On the preparations of the Indian Hemp, or Gunjah*; London, *Provinces Medical Journal* No. 123; February 1843.]

Indian hemp is grown freely in the native states to the south of Raipur and smuggling it is both easy and profitable. In the treatment of *Convulsions*, the use of dry cannabis herb in smoke form, is popular among the traditional healers of Chhattisgarh. The herb is put on the fire and patients are advised to inhale the fumes. In rural India, the inhalation of pungent smells is a method used to abort on-going convulsions. A popular method across the country is to smell footwear or onion and garlic. The tribals of Chhattisgarh burn insects and inhale the fumes to stop epileptic fits. Caterpillars, bed bugs and earthworms are dried and stored in jars for this purpose by traditional healers. Foul smells are considered effective in suppressing convulsion. At times, soil contaminated with the urine of a wild boar is used as treatment. Since the oral administration of drugs is not possible during an acute attack, most herbal medicines are used as nasal drops.

Ayurvedic medicines are available for over-the-counter sale with, (in general perception), less toxicity and better tolerability. The *brahmi* plant is traditionally used as a nerve tonic, an antiepileptic and anti-asthmatic drug; however, a very high dosage of *brahmi* is required to suppress seizures. It has been proposed to use it as an adjuvant to anti-epileptic drugs for its inherent cognitive benefits, especially in childhood epilepsy. Barbiturates were used for many years for psychiatric and epileptic patients. *Phenobarbiturates* were followed by *phenytoin sodium*. The combination of these two drugs is still popular in rural India as an effective medication and distributed by doctors and quacks alike. It was extensively used by an agency and attracted a number of drug refractory epileptics from rural India to Rishikesh, where this combination was given along with herbal preparations. In fact, similar practices are observed all over the Indian subcontinent.

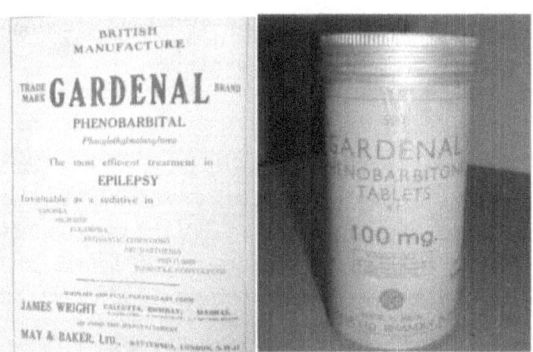

FIG 35: Drug to survive & to die. May & Baker Co. introduced *Gardenal* (Phenobarbitone), used for epilepsy and multiple other indications, to calm patients. Crude but very effective as a medicinal pill for humans and animals, long-acting barbiturates are used for *euthanasia*.

The chronic side-effects of *phenytoin* (e.g. disfiguring gum swelling, coarsening of facial features, drunkard gait and slurred speech), became all too common in outdoor units, and the drug destroyed the looks of many faces. *Gum hyperplasia* is known to have occurred in a substantial number of adults who consumed *phenytoin sodium* for the treatment of epilepsy. Young age at the time of *phenytoin* prescription, poor dental hygiene, and unmonitored high blood levels from the drug, all contributed to *dental hyperplasia*. *Hyperplasia* is most prominent over dental plaque in experimental animals like the stump-tail monkey (*Macaca Arctoides*). Exposure to *phenytoin* and poor dental hygiene lead to tooth area exposure in animals, which can be prevented by the simple local application of *chlorhexidine* solution (mouthwash). At times, the entire tooth is engulfed by the growth of the gums. It takes about three months to develop and subsides rapidly on cessation of the drug.

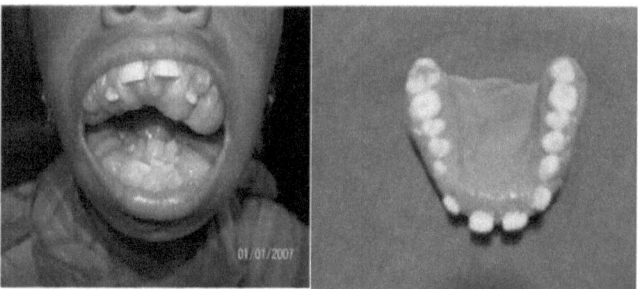

FIG 36: Devil's denture. *Phenytoin*-induced massive gum swelling in a patient on long-standing therapy for epilepsy. (Courtesy: Drs Suneel Vyas, Rahul Shrivastava, YP Nagraj). The mould of the removable upper denture (left), is to be noted. An epileptic patient, after seven years of *phenytoin* therapy, showed gum growth along the concave inner surface of the upper dental plate as well as buried teeth.

At times, *purple glove syndrome* (PGS), occurred due to the intravenous administration of *phenytoin*. The tissue necrosis is caused by drug leakage into the subcutaneous plain. PGS is not rare amongst elderly patients or individuals who receive large, multiple doses of intravenous *phenytoin sodium*. Severe cases may require surgical intervention (e.g. surgery of the skin and underlying tissue, called *fasciotomy*) to relieve pressure and restore blood flow.

NOTE

1. Very striking cases have been published, both in America and in Africa, of the complete cure of epilepsy following the bites of poisonous snakes in which, though the patients were made very ill, the amount of venom injected was not sufficient to cause death. There are a number of records of patients treated by the injection of snake venom in which it is claimed that long-standing epilepsy has been cured. [Elliot, R.H. *Treatment of Epilepsy by Snake Venom; BMJ*; December 1934, 1073]

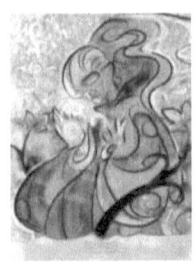

22 SEIZURES OF DIFFERENT KINDS

CONVULSIVE THERAPY FOR SCHIZOPHRENIA
This patient had several courses of pyrexial therapy (sulfosin) *with no apparent improvement. Shock therapy* (cardiazol) *commenced on 2 March 1938. He had six intravenous injections ranging from 4 to 6 c.cm. of a 10 per cent cardiazol solution. Good reactions were noted; however, the intravenous route was difficult. A seventh and subsequent convulsions was induced by the intramuscular route (6 c.cm. of a 30 per cent cardiazol solution). In all, fourteen convulsions were induced. The patient was greatly improved socially...* [Taylor, M. *Convulsion Therapy in Schizophrenia; Indian Medical Gazette;* October 1938]

In earlier times, convulsions were induced to treat madness. It was observed that in a number of schizophrenics, remissions followed epileptic attacks. In 1930, Muller reported two cases of *catatonic schizophrenia* that recovered after having *epileptiform* fits. While working in the laboratory of the Royal State Mental Hospitals in Budapest, Dr Ladislaus von Meduna, believed that in the development of schizophrenia and epilepsy, there existed a fundamental biological antagonism, which could, by artificial means, be made to serve therapeutic ends. He first tried intramuscular injections of camphor in oil, but these had to be discontinued because of the large doses required. Eventually, *pentylene tetrazol*, known as *cardiazol* (Knoll), proved to be more practical and effective. The drug is soluble in water and can be used intravenously, intramuscularly and subcutaneously. When used in the right quantity and with sufficient rapidity, a typical epileptic convulsion is produced 10 to 90 seconds after the injection. In cases treated by the intramuscular route, the time varies from 5 to 90 minutes after the injection. It was found that a combination of *insulin* and *cardiazol* gave good results when *cardiazol* alone failed to produce convulsions. The practice was to administer 20 to 50 units of *insulin* subcutaneously two hours before the *cardiazol* injection. During the first six months of 1938, 26 patients were treated at the Ranchi Mental Hospital. Of the 26 cases, 11 made complete recoveries, while 10 showed improvement, and 5 showed no improvement.

PREGNANCY-RELATED SEIZURES

At 1:15 AM, while a patient was being comforted by her sister – the nurse also by the bedside – she started to talk incoherently. A general convulsive shiver was observed; her complexion immediately assumed a livid hue and her eyes became fixed, pupils dilated. Her breathing was short and jerky and her pulse barely perceptible. Uterine action ceased entirely, and death appeared imminent. The symptoms rapidly passed into a deep coma, the conjunctive failing to respond to touch, or the pupils to light, leaving little room to doubt that one of the most formidable of puerperal complications had supervened in the form of cerebral apoplexy. [McCabe, D.A. *Puerperal convulsions*; Indian Medical Gazette; August 1905]

The convulsions during the final stages of pregnancy signify a serious underlying disorder and disturb all the joy otherwise attached to it. *Puerperal convulsions* were considered a different class of epileptic fit, that affected the healthiest women more often. Symptoms of cerebral congestion (*cerebral oedema*), preceded the attacks. Hissing respiration was thought to be characteristic, and it was noted that fits struck in rapid succession. McCabe (1905), classified *puerperal convulsions* in three different etiological groups: *hyperaemia* secondary to circulatory disturbances; *anaemia* as in cases of extreme haemorrhage; and lastly, *toxaemia* of pregnancy.

In the past, these paroxysms were often fatal. *Puerperal convulsions* required different management. Bazaar medicine recommended the application of turpentine or mustard to the extremities and evaporating lotion to the head, while camphor and calomel or borax and cinnamon pills, were given internally. A turpentine enema was also thought to be useful.

Convulsions soon after delivery, in the absence of *hypertension* and *eclampsia*, may suggest a venous stroke resulting from *thrombosis,* in sluggishly flowing blood in the cerebral veins and sinuses. Convulsions frequently occur at the beginning and are associated with raised intracranial tension, altered sensorium and even death. *Puerperal venous thrombosis* is said to be precipitated by a fast maintained for at least three days by the mother of a new-born child. The new mother is given jaggery and herbs boiled in water for three days. On the fifth day after childbirth, which is marked by celebrations, the mother is fed dried lentil balls and other foods. The tradition of fasting has become less common, but most new mothers have serum B-12 deficiency and *anaemia*.

Mackie (1929), described this form of *anaemia* under the title 'malignant anaemia of the tropics'. It was common amongst both men and women in Bombay. Two years later, Wills (1931), showed that *macrocytic anaemia,* which was particularly common amongst pregnant women and was curable by the oral administration of *autolysed yeast* (marmite). She called the condition 'tropical macrocytic anaemia' and considered it primarily a nutritional condition. *Tropical macrocytic anaemia* was common in India where the diet was grossly deficient in extrinsic factors. One study demonstrated that among vegetarians, it developed at the rate of 54.1 per 1000 per year, while not at all among non-vegetarians. It worsens during pregnancy and rapidly responds to supplements of liver abstract or marmite.

Toxaemia with *albuminuria* was called renal convulsion. This distinct type of convulsion is associated with higher mortality. There are ancient accounts of *eclampsia* and complications of pregnancy and childbirth in Indian literature. In the *Atharva-veda* and *Sushruta* texts, there are references to the use of amulets in pregnancy to prevent convulsions in childbirth. The aetiology of *eclampsia* and seizure is poorly understood, and there is considerable disagreement with regard to the ideal anticonvulsant for the prevention and control of these seizures.

She slept only however for about one hour, and on waking at 9 pm was seized with an epileptiform convulsion; this fit was followed by others throughout the night, and when seen at 8 am on 22nd October, she had eight fits, lasting from two to three minutes each. The patient was now in a semi-conscious condition and complaining of intense headache and pain in the back of the neck. The tongue was swollen and badly bitten, the respirations hurried and shallow, and the pulse feeble, 120 to the minute, urine scanty and loaded with albumin. [Barry, C. Notes on a case of puerperal eclampsia treated by hypodermic injection of morphia; Indian Medical Gazette; February 1904]

India contributes about a quarter of global maternal deaths. WHO defines maternal mortality as the death of a woman during pregnancy and the first 42 days after the birth of a child, due to events linked with pregnancy. The life expectancy in prehistoric times was low for women between 25-40 years, who often suffered from malnutrition and died during childbirth. The country has a disturbingly high maternal mortality rate (MMR). Pre-existing malnutrition, early marriage, prolonged fasting after childbirth, all contributed to illness. In the Hindu religion, woman were considered impure during childbirth, which resulted in neglect of the problem. A woman's life was not precious in the harem either. A slave-girl or concubine was attended poorly during childbirth. A female *jarrah* (surgeon), attached to the *Shafa- Khanah* (hospital), of the palace, performed minor surgeries. The sick lady was not taken out of the palace even when medication failed and she required major surgery. Often, she eventually succumbed to her illness. Pre or post-natal care of slave-girls or concubines was not of much consequence and they were easily replaced in the harem.

The only assistance during childbirth was provided by indigenous *dai*s across the country. These country midwives acquired some skill from other *dai*s but were completely illiterate about hygiene The British perceived the practices of the *dai*s as barbaric and primitive; and they slowly started showing interest in improving midwifery in India. Evangelistic missions began work related to healthcare of Indian women. Gradually hospitals run by women missionaries became popular places to deliver babies in the remote corners of India.

The Queen's interest in the health of native women, was stimulated by a letter from the Maharani of Panna, who was treated by Dr. Elizabeth Bielby, a professor of midwifery in Lahore. Thereafter, Queen Victoria communicated to Lady Dufferin the urgent need to provide female medical professionals to serve Indian women. Much attention was paid to women's welfare under the aegis of successive Vicerines. Indians appreciated the benefits of improved childbirth techniques that resulted in fewer dead infants and women surviving difficult pregnancies. As the Indian princes saw the pain and suffering of childbirth reduced, they were impressed enough by Western medicine to entrust the lives of their own wives and concubines to the safety of Western medical procedure. Further training programmes were started for native *dai*s during the British Raj. However, the improved obstetrical services, so important for safe delivery, had not reached rural India, and many deliveries were still conducted at home, assisted by poorly trained *dai*s.

A child's brain also suffers during difficult deliveries. Lack of blood supply and oxygen to the developing brain, at times results in gross destruction of brain substances that is replaced by fluid-filled cavities. A syndrome of *multi-cystic encephalomalacia* may then set in, which is characterised by a small and deformed skull, poor visual and auditory attention, decreased movements of limbs, and frequent convulsions. The limbs only move in jerks. The syndrome could well be a terminal affliction and there is no definite prognosis as to how long the child would survive, lying on a bed without attaining further development.

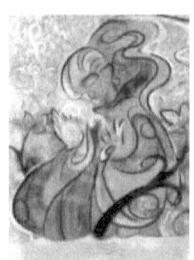

23 CHILDREN & GENES

CHILDREN OF THE SUN
God blessed them with a single sickle cell gene (*sickle cell trait*), that confers relative protection against *falciparum malaria* during a critical phase in early childhood, and they are less likely to die from malaria. These children survived, married and expanded their families. Now many of the children with Sickler genetic characteristics have a pair of *sickle cell genes* and the *lethal sickle cell disease.*

GENETIC CONSTITUTION
The migration of large sections of the population who work as labourers, is common in the state of Chhattisgarh; but they come back for social purposes and marry each other (only those from the same caste and from nearby villages). Marriages bereft of free selection and constrained by endogamous restrictions, increase the chances of transmitting characteristics, which creates localised pockets in the rural population with the same genetic disorders.

Sickle cell anaemia is one of the most prevalent genetic disorders in Chhattisgarh. The disorder is prevalent in all 18 districts of the state and is alarming in 10 of them. Approximately 9-10 % of the population have been found to be either sickle cell carriers or sufferers of the disease. In such cases, peculiarly elongated and sickle-shaped red corpuscles are found in the blood. The low oxygen-carrying capacity of these deformed red cells causes *anaemia* and other problems.

Those with the severe disease do not survive childhood. They often have retardation of growth and complicated lives with painful crises and recurrent infections, and require repeated blood transfusions. Those who survive with the milder form, in a carrier state, have what is called the *sickle cell trait*. One may identify the sickle cell trait sometimes in a long, slender body frame. Problems arise when two persons with the trait marry and produce a child with *sickle cell disease*.

The first formal recognition of *sickle cell disease* was in a 20-year-old medical student from Grenada, in the West Indies, who was attending school in Chicago. A review of the first four cases reported in the United States, noted that all were of African ancestry. This high prevalence in equatorial Africa and its predominance among populations of African origin in the Caribbean and the United States, led to the belief that the sickle cell gene was confined to people of African origin and in some way racially linked. Those who so believed, thought that the most significant feature of *sickle cell anaemia* was the fact that its occurrence depended entirely on the presence of Negro blood, albeit in extremely small quantities. There are two principal determinants of the present worldwide distribution of the sickle cell gene: movements of affected populations and mutation. The Atlantic slave trade accounted for the movement of large populations carrying the sickle cell gene from the coastal areas of west and central Africa to the Caribbean Islands, the United States and South America.

As regards the Indian scenario, Lehmann and Miss Cutbush discovered *sickle cell haemoglobin* in the Nilgiri hills in south India, in 1952. Incidentally, Lehman's group also first recognised the sickle cell gene in Saudi Arabia. The abnormal haemoglobin remained his major interest. He travelled all over the world collecting blood samples and identified a number of human haemoglobin variants. He realised that the distribution of abnormal haemoglobin among different populations could provide invaluable anthropological information. He started searching for the lost link between south India, Arabia and Africa. F. C. Hoyte, surgical registrar, lost his life on 7 July 1958, at 32 years of age, when climbing in the Karakoram range of the Himalayas. He collected specimens for the examination of abnormal haemoglobin in Sind and from the isolated Hunza tribe. The specimens he collected from Sind have supplied an important anthropological link between south India, Arabia and Africa, in the form of the first example of sickle cell trait from west Pakistan.

The Anthropological Survey of India has coordinated extensive studies indicating the sickle cell gene to be widespread throughout much of central India, reaching sickle cell trait frequencies of 20 to 30 % in some areas. It forms a belt across central parts of India, touching important ports in the coastal states of Gujarat and Andhra Pradesh, where some migration of the population took place through the established silk and spice routes, but not in the magnitude discovered in central India. The likely explanation is that, either the sickle cell gene developed independently in the two areas, or that the peoples of both areas, with common non-African ancestors, inherited it. The *Asian haplotype* appears to be consistently associated with high levels of *haemoglobin of foetal origin* (HbF) with a lower *haemolytic* rate. The clinical consequences are generally a milder course of illness with fewer *vaso-occlusive* episodes and a greater persistence of *splenomegaly*.

TRIBE OF BALD LADIES

The typical face and baldness in its ageing females suggest that the *Agharia* Patel community is from the bordering region of Chhattisgarh and Orissa. Dr Vinita Naik considered the *Agharias* of Chhattisgarh and adjoining Orissa, Madhya Pradesh and Chhota Nagpur, to be *Jats*, who had migrated from the region around Agra. Recent research on the *Agharias*, particularly the distribution of their chromosomes and blood groups, suggests that they are native to the northern Gangetic plains. They have two main sub-divisions, the *Bade* or superior *Agharias*, and the *Chhota*, or inferior/mixed

Agharias. In different settlements, they are further sub-divided as *Ratanpuria, Phuljharia* and *Raigarhia* (i.e. those living around Ratanpur, Phuljhar and Raigarh).

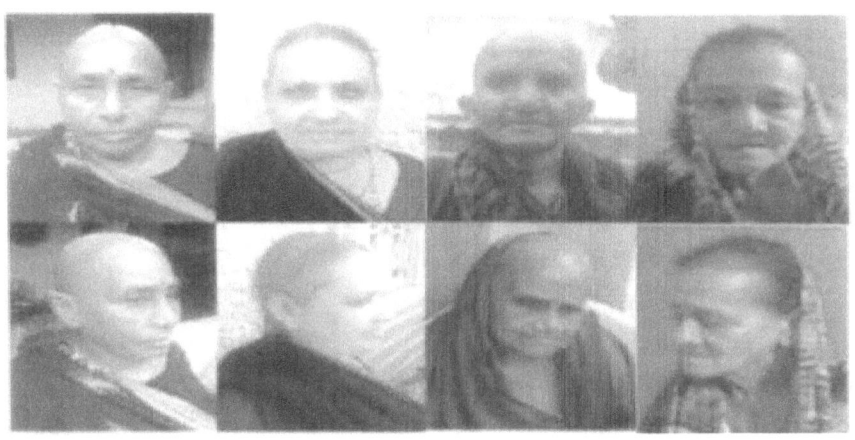

FIG 37: Progressive baldness of elderly *Agharia* Patel women.

The females gradually lose their long hair by the time they reach middle age. Their traditions (i.e. of tying their hair too tightly with a comb and covering the head with a *saree*, which produces constant rubbing, and pulling out their own hair), are blamed for their progressive baldness. The widening of the central parting in the hair appears most noticeably in the mid-frontal scalp.

Patterned balding in women differs (in terms of age of onset, rate of progression and pattern), from male balding. Often, hair loss in women is not confined to the crown and may extend from ear to ear. To date, there have been no comparable genetic studies on female pattern hair loss.

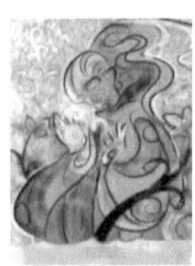

24 Deficient Diet

No preventive campaign against malaria, against tuberculosis or against leprosy, no maternity relief or child welfare activities are likely to achieve any great success unless those responsible recognise the vital importance of this factor of defective nutrition and from the very start give it their most serious attention. Abundant supplies of quinine and multiplication of tuberculosis hospitals, sanatoria, leprosy colonies and maternity and child-welfare centres are no doubt desirable, if not essential, but none of these go to the root of matter. The first essentials for the prevention of disease are a higher standard of health, a better physique and a great power of resistance to infection. These can only be attained if the food of people is such as will give all the physiological and nutritional requirements of the human frame. [Sir Alexander Russell. *Public Health Commissioner Report* (1935)]

The late 18th and 19th centuries saw frequent famines in the Indian subcontinent. The British government was severely criticised for the inadequate measures taken to combat famine. In the British era (1770–1947), over 50 million lives perished in India in about 40 famine outbreaks involving different geographical distributions. During the Rajputana famine, between 1868 and 1870, 1.5 million inhabitants of Marwar died, and another 1.5 million were said to have emigrated (approximately a million along with their cattle). The Famine Commissioner for the Government of India, Richard Temple, decided the wage for relief work would be was one pound of grain plus one anna (6.25 paisa) for a man, with small reductions for a woman or child. The relief programme was later called 'Temple

Wages'. Famine frequently hit Raipur on account of rice crop failure. The mortality during famine rose from 41 per mile in 1896 to 81 for the year 1897. Despite major crop failure, the minor millet crops of *Kodo* and *Kutki* often survived. The forest tribes thrived on it and were little affected during famines. Although *Kodo* millet is still under cultivation as an auxiliary food grain in different parts of Chhattisgarh, in earlier times it was a main crop in the tribal belt.

Lathyrism is an ancient disorder connected to war, famine and pestilence. An early classic account of the disease was provided by Sleeman in 1833: *During these three years (1829–1831), the teor, or what in the other parts of India is called kesari (the Lathyrus Sativus of botanists), a kind of wild vetch, which, though not sown itself, is left carelessly to grow among the wheat and other grain, and given in the green and dry state to cattle, remained uninjured, and thrived with great luxuriance. In 1831, they reaped a rich crop of it from blighted wheat fields and subsisted upon its grain during that and the following years, giving the stalks and leaves only to their cattle. In 1833, the sad effects of this food began to manifest themselves. The younger part of the population of this and surrounding villages, from the age of thirty downwards, began to be deprived of the use of their limbs below the waist by paralytic strokes... No person once attacked had been found to recover the use of the limbs affected, and my tent was surrounded by great numbers of the youth in different stages of the disease...*

Lathyrism was especially prevalent in the Central Province, where epidemics lasted from 1896 until 1902. In India, the cultivation of *L. sativus* was prohibited in Allahabad in 1870, because of successive epidemics reported by Irving. In north Rewa in 1921, it was estimated that 6 % of the total population of about a million people, were affected. The then Maharaja of Rewa State, passed an order on 29 November 1907, prohibiting the cultivation of *L. sativus*. *Lathyrism* is still encountered in central India, eastern UP and Bangladesh. An epidemiological survey conducted by Dwivedi and Mishra, in the Indian districts of Durg, Rajnandgaon and Raipur in the 1980s, discovered nine new cases. The sufferers consumed grass pea in a particular manner: *The Indian staple* ghotu, *prepared by cooking a mixture of grass pea and rice...precipitated* lathyrism *more rapidly than* chapatti, *the unleavened bread form.* All nine cases gave histories of getting the disease about 20 days after consuming *ghotu*, containing mainly *lathyrus* flour with small quantities of rice. In 1984, two cases were recorded from Raipur.

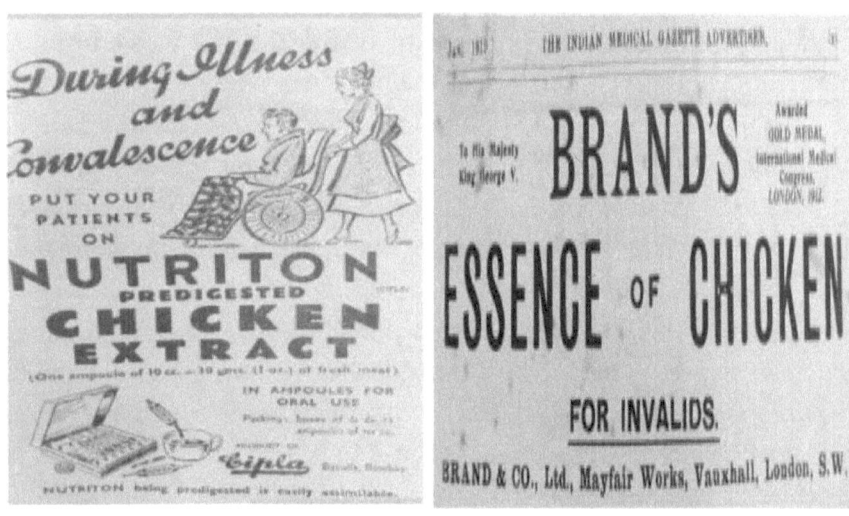

FIG 38: Food supplements for non-vegetarians: Chicken supplements prescribed for faster recovery from debility. **Another advertisement:** A chicken nutritional supplement for invalids.

Multiple nutritional problems existed in India, which gradually became less common due to improved diet; these included *beriberi*, a disease of the rice eater; *pellagra*, a disease of the maize eater; and *kwashiorkor* and *marasmus*, associated with lack of protein. On the other hand, European soldiers also lost weight considerably, their strength and health being impaired by heat and illness. Multiple food supplementations and tonics flooded the market to replenish their strength and vigour, mostly derived from meat. Extractions of beef in alcohol, beef juices and beef tea, pre-digested chicken extract, cod liver emulsion and pancreatic emulsions, were the sources of potent substances. Highly concentrated, strength-giving tonics were prepared by adding iron, combining quinine with beef extract dissolved in pure medicinal wine, or cod liver oil emulsified with malt, etc. Most of these were unsuited to the strictly vegetarian Hindu population.

As noted by Satnam (translated by Vishav Bharti): *In the tribal belt, proper food is not available year-round. They dry small amount of fish for the lean period. When fish is available, there is plenty of bamboo, too, but the bamboo dries up and hardens before the fish disappear. Therefore, they eat the bamboo instead. When winter ends, they begin collecting wild roots for survival.*

Lack of sleep with vivid dreams and various psychosomatic disturbances appeared in a Vitamin B-12-deficient state. The Jain scholars, due to their severe dietary restrictions, often suffer from chronic anaemia and B-12 deficiency. Once they develop symptoms of deficiency, it is impossible to treat them, as supplementation by allopathic drugs is still not allowed in certain sects of Jainism. Many times, Vitamin B-complex deficiency results in an acute burning sensation in the hands and feet. In the majority of cases, it is so severe that it prevents the patient from walking and frequently necessitates the administration of narcotics to produce sleep. The affected patients try all sorts of physical treatments for relief from the pain that keeps them awake night after night.

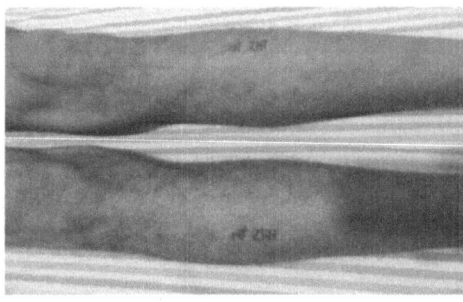

FIG 39: Branding of the name of God, on both legs, for relief of neuropathic pain.

J. Grierson, a British Medical officer in the Indian Army, read a paper in Calcutta in 1825. About a century later, the paper was referred to in 1946, by Gopalan, an Indian nutritional biochemist, who described a certain condition in females between the ages 20 and 40 years, among the poor in south India. It was effectively treated with *calcium pantothenate* (B-5) and is now known as the *Grierson-Gopalan syndrome* or 'burning feet' syndrome. A similar syndrome was described by J. Pagein, in 1825, the same year as the publication of Grierson's paper, regarding observations made among male prisoners of war in the Far East, all of whom subsisted mainly on rice gruel and vegetables. The disease was also fairly common in the Malay Peninsula, chiefly in labourers in coffee plantations, usually with a 'pins and needles' sensation affecting the soles of the feet, which prevented them from working in the fields on hot days. Gerrard called it *Erythromelalgia Tropica*. *Erythromelalgia* is a clinical syndrome defined by a history of red, hot extremities. The symptoms include flushing of the affected extremities, which become very painful and sometimes disabling.

A tropical atmosphere and rice diet appeared to be the common factors in all such syndromes seen so frequently in Chhattisgarh, where rice is the main staple food. The inhabitants eat rice in many forms, from freshly steamed rice served with lots of spices to stale (*basi*) rice served with salt and onions. People eat rice in the morning, afternoon and at night, and often spend their entire lives growing and selling the grain. Rice governs their lives. Bazaar medicine recommends the application of *henna*, a shrub with small green leaves used to colour the hands and hair red, on the soles of the feet, to reduce the burning sensation: *The leaves of this common Indian shrub, henna, are almost universally used throughout the East for staining the nails and hair and are well worthy of a trial in the treatment of that troublesome and painful affliction of the natives called burning of the feet. For this purpose, the fresh leaves should be beaten into a paste with vinegar or lime juice and applied as a poultice to the soles of the feet.*

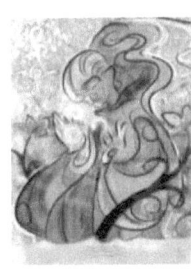

25 ADDICTIONS

When, therefore, these 5,000 British medical practitioners signed a petition that Her Majesty's subjects in India should be deprived of their liberty to indulge in the use of opium, whilst they jealously guard the liberty to indulge in alcohol for their own people, it could only have been from the strong conviction that the opium habit was incomparably more vicious, degrading and mischievous to the mind and body than the alcoholic habit.
[*Crombie and the Opium Question; Indian Medical Gazette*; Nov. 1893]

SEDATIVES

The use of recreational drugs resulted in the discovery of some of the earlier medicines for neurological disorders, aimed at calming violent headaches, convulsions, psychotic episodes and tetanic spasms. Indians had been aware of some of these herbal sedatives from ancient times. Mahatma Gandhi reportedly chewed the root of *R. serpentina* to help achieve a state of philosophic detachment while meditating. Indians also looked for aphrodisiac properties in this medicinal group, apart from its tranquilising properties. In ancient India, alcohol and smoke were frequently mixed with herbal medicine for extra strength and other benefits.

The British recorded stories of a plant known to science as *Datura metel*, related to the nightshades in India. They described its flower as so powerful that its fragrance alone would fell passers-by. *Datura* attained a negative reputation as a roadside poison. A professional poisoner used its powdered seeds mixed with sweetmeats and distributed it as *prasad* at a temple. Sometimes wheat flour was mixed with *datura* flour; or the distilled essence of *datura* was used with sugar. This poison is still frequently used as a drug, especially for long bus or train journeys, and not with the intention of destroying life. In earlier times death did occur but infrequently. Dr Burton Brown, recorded 20 deaths from 92 cases of *datura* poisoning in Lahore, while Bombay recorded 24 deaths from 138 cases.

POPPY

I have no hesitation in recommending the habitual use of opium in European children during the period of dentition and whereas formerly many children used to die in my practice from enteritis, which is the scourge of European infant life in India, now I rarely if ever lose a case from this disease. [Evidence given by Surgeon – Lieutenant Colonel Lawrie E. before the Royal Commission on Opium on 4 Jan. 1894]

In all probability, opium was introduced into India by nomadic Arab traders and invaders. The drug was extensively taken by mouth for its euphoric effects in the times of Akbar, as shown by the reference made to it by Abul-Fazl in his book, *Ain-i-akbari*. By the 11th century, it was recognised for its recreational and aphrodisiac qualities. British India established a monopoly over opium production in Bengal in 1793, with most of it being shipped to Canton, China.

Indians were moderate users of opium as compared to the Chinese. In Punjab, Sikh men who consumed opium, were capable of withstanding a great deal of fatigue. A small amount of opium stopped all cravings for food for days. Its use was thus a means of keeping the body and soul together during periods of chronic starvation. If opium was taken after the age of 45, it secured a longer life. For younger people, opium was used as an aphrodisiac. It was a time-honoured practice of Indian mothers to give their babies opium as a sleeping solution. Opium was given almost universally to children for teething and diarrhea, without causing any harm.

The poor man rather prefers to have a glass of country wine, 'sharab' , but he cannot afford it; as it now costs ten annas per bottle of twenty-four ounces, and it takes half a bottle to 'put him forrard*' while he feels at peace with all the world after eating a halfpenny worth of opium.
[* *'Forrard' = Frontward*]

Ethnicity and the Chinese influence, were considered responsible for the higher incidence of opium smoking in Assam and Burma as compared to the other parts of India. The high incidence in the Central Provinces was, however, puzzling. Opium smoking spread to certain districts inhabited by aboriginal tribes, such as Raipur, Balaghat, Bilaspur and Mandla. An estimate of *madak* smokers in these districts in 1933, was 1707, 868, 490 and 400 respectively. Raipur was even worse affected than the notorious Narshingpur sub-division, where the number was 1500.

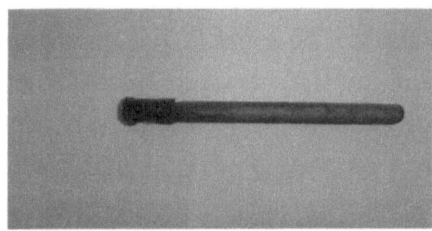

FIG 40: *Madak* **opium smoking pipe.** Indians preferred to eat opium rather than to smoke it – a culture adopted from Persia (Courtesy: Dr Inam MD)

CANNABIS

The recreational use of Indian hemp was practiced in India from time immemorial and found a place in the religious and social observances of the Hindus. It was a great favourite of God *Shiva* and his followers, called *Shaivites*. Hemp was viewed as promoting success and strength. It caused a reeling gait, apart from being laughter-inducing and an aphrodisiac.

The narcotic product of the hemp plant (*Cannabis sativa / indica*), that is consumed in India, falls under three main categories: *ganja* (dried flowering top of female hemp plant), *charas* (resin) and *bhang* (dried leaves). *Ganja* was popular in Assam, Bengal,

Madras, Bombay and the Central Provinces. *Charas* was mainly derived from Central Asia and mostly consumed in northern India, while *bhang* was consumed all over India. *Majum* was the stronger preparation made of Indian hemp leaves, milk, clarified butter, poppy seeds, flowers of the thorn apple, *nux vomica* powder and sugar. It was only when a powerful narcotic was required that all these ingredients were used. In 1893, a commission was appointed to enquire into the production of hemp drugs and their effects on society. The commission showed that *bhang* is almost without exception harmless when used in moderation and not as hurtful as intemperate indulgence in alcohol. Between the years 1880 and 1900, hemp drugs and country spirits contributed equally towards revenue through excise duties.

In Ayurveda, cannabis is added to destroy phlegm, expel flatulence, induce costiveness, sharpen the memory, increase eloquence, excite the appetite and act as a general tonic. The Persian writer of the *Mukzun-ul-Udwieh*, waxes eloquent on the versatile qualities of hemp leaves: *The leaves make a good snuff for deterging the brain; the juice of the leaves applied to the head as a wash removes dandruff and vermin; drops of the juice thrown into the ear allay pain and destroy worms or insects. It checks diarrhoea, is useful in gonorrhoea, restrains seminal secretions and is diuretic.*

William Brooke O' Shaughnessy, Professor of Chemistry and *materia medica* at Calcutta Medical College, picked Indian cannabis to introduce from Indian traditional medicine into Western medicinal prescriptions. Apart from headaches, he also used it to treat childhood convulsions, relieve painful spasms in cases of tetanus, rabies, rheumatism and cholera. Unlike opium, it does not cause constipation and increases the appetite. Indian cannabis was considered an effective agent for treating epilepsy. The world is now opening up again to the use of cannabis and marijuana for treating *epilepsy, multiple sclerosis, amyotrophic lateral sclerosis* and *refractory pain.*

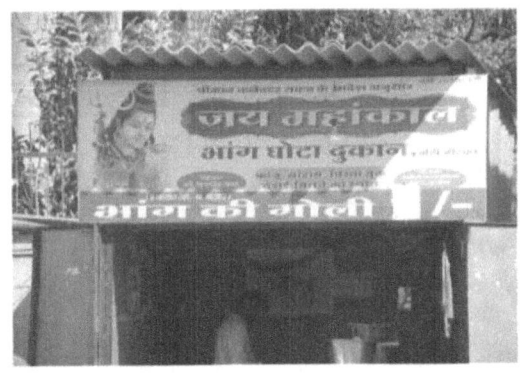

FIG 41: **Official Indian hemp shop**, near Indore airport.

OTHER SUBSTANCE ABUSE

Seekers of cheap addiction often resort to patterned use (or rather misuse), of opiate analgesics, codeine-containing cough syrups, high alcohol-containing local herbal tonics, painkiller balms, or even inhaling non-medical substances like glues and paints, for such irregular purposes as inducing mood-alteration, stimulation, sedation, hallucination etc. For example, groups of young individuals typically consume capsules of *spasmo-proxyvon* (SP) to precipitate seizures for pleasure. The Wockhardt India Company markets the drug in India. The combination of drugs includes *dicyclomine hydrochloride, propoxyphene napsylate* and *acetaminophen* to provide symptomatic relief from abdominal pain. It is popularly known as SP or blue cap, in the market and is an over-the-counter drug. Youths purchase the drug and consume it at regular intervals. Seizures are precipitated after the consumption of 8-10 capsules. These seizures are generalised tonic-clonic in nature and occur within a few hours of consuming a higher than usual dose. As seizure precipitation is often a dose-related event, addicts often consume five or six capsules together in the morning and take a top-up dose after two or three hours, to precipitate a seizure by the afternoon. Some addicts have developed a relative tolerance and consume over 100 capsules a day.

A disproportionately high rate of epileptic seizures has been noted in patients who abuse *dextropropoxyphene* (DPP). Results of one study showed that of 312 patients who abused DPP, 63 (20.2 %) had epileptic seizures related to DPP in contrast to 0.4–4.2 % amongst other *opioid* users.

ALCOHOL

The ancient Aryan invaders brought the art of brewing alcoholic drinks to India around 2000 BC. They used a beverage called *soma*. *Soma* was a drink from the *Vedic* period, possibly brewed from plants like hemp, *ephedra* or *sarcostemma*. The medical treatise of *Charaka* and *Sushruta* mentioned multiple types of medicinal alcoholic drinks. A detailed description of the use of alcoholic beverages is found in Kautilya's *Arthashastra* (3rd century BC). The manufacture and sale of alcoholic drinks was a state monopoly. The drinks were made mostly from the fermentation of rice, barley, fruit juices and beans; grape-based wines were imported from Afghanistan. Palm-wine drinking is predominant in the Afro-Asian culture. *Taadi*, distilled from the coconut palm, remained a favourite drink in south India. Edward Terry, during his travels in India between 1616 and 1619, commented on a liquor called *taadi* (toddy): *[I]t is a piercing medicinal drink, if taken early and moderately as some have found by happy experience, thereby eased from their torture inflicted by that shame of physicians and tyrant of all maladies, the stone.*

Arrac is a distilled and stronger version of *taadi*. *Arrac* was said to be good for abdominal pain and constipation, and was loved by the British troops in India. There was a strong belief among the hill tribes of India, that fermented beverages were a necessity to survive the damp and cold and that they were prophylactics against malaria. Multiple variants of domestic liquor are consumed in Chhattisgarh. *Mahua* is a fermented drink obtained from the flowers of the *Madhuca longifolia* and *Sulfi*, a palm wine extracted from the fishtail palm. The *Mahua* tree flowers in February and March. The flowers are collected by women and children and hundreds can be seen leaving their villages in the early dawn to collect the fallen flowers.

In Chhattisgarh, the number of *Sulfi* trees in a house is an indicator of the wealth and prosperity of the household. Doctors in the 18th century, considered wine one of the medicines for treating tropical fevers. Europeans in the tropics would drink more alcohol than at home, partly for social reasons and partly due to the mistaken belief that alcohol was necessary for health in the tropics. Large shipments of wines from England and France were regularly dispatched to Calcutta. The first distillery was established at Kanpur in 1805, and by the end of the 19th century, a number of breweries in India produced beer, rum, gin and whisky. The drinking habits and tastes of the native gentry were gradually transformed to include foreign liquor, Indian-made foreign liquor and domestic liquor alike.

Certain toxic chemicals and pesticides, when added to distilled drinks, strengthen them. At times, an unpleasant burning sensation develops in the palms and soles, due to *arsenic neuropathy*. More problems are generated from the consumption of bootlegged alcohol. Illicit liquor has been responsible for killing many and rendering others blind. These accidents occur in states where alcohol is prohibited or areas ridden with poverty or on the outskirts of metro cities. In Gujarat, over 100 people died from drinking illegal bootleg alcohol, in one incident alone, as alcohol is banned in the state. Recently, a large number of deaths were registered in Calcutta due to the consumption of illicit liquor.

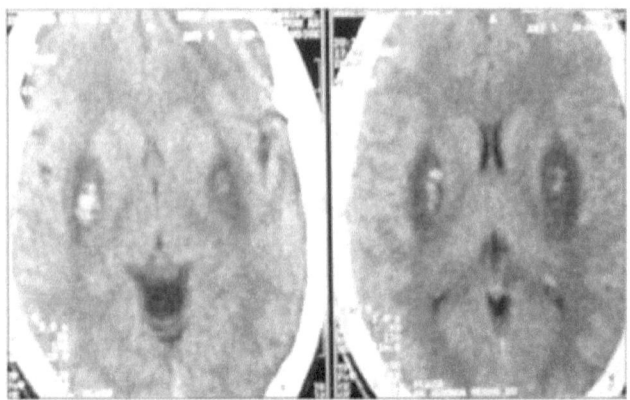

FIG 42: Happy & Sad Face. A 45-year-old man was hospitalised with complaints of altered consciousness and recurrent vomiting. He had consumed a denatured surgical spirit bought from the hospital. Two days later, he recovered, though he was blind. Both his *basal ganglion nuclei* had bled and generated scars as a marker of denatured spirit (*methanol*) *toxic encephalopathy*. Weirdly enough, the lesion appeared as laughing and crying faces on CT-scan sections.

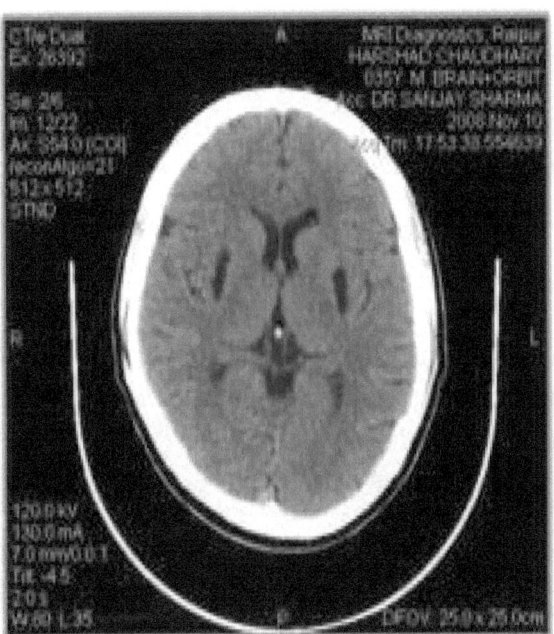

FIG 43: HC, a 34-year-old male, was admitted to the emergency department with recurrent vomiting, *altered sensorium* and *metabolic acidosis*. Further history revealed consumption of a bottle of vodka followed by two bottles of perfume, as no other *ethanol* was available to him on the evening of 31 December 2008. His *metabolic acidosis* was corrected in the ICU. On regaining sensation, he noted profound blindness. When examined later, he was able to count fingers placed up to three feet from his right eye and up to one foot from his left, and bilateral pale optic disks on both sides. His CT-Head repeated a year later on 10 November 2009, showed *bilateral symmetrical hypodensity* involving the *globus* and in the putamen nucleus deep inside the brain. In fact, often in such cases, the initial CT scan is normal, and several days may elapse before the lesions become evident.

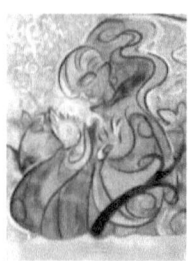

26 SEX & LONGEVITY

I know no association of Ayurvedic physicians that protest against or endeavour to check this ceaseless flow of immorality which is sapping Indian manhood and making of many old men monsters, living merely to satisfy their lust. [Mahatma Gandhi]

The Persian influence brought into prominence yet another group of medicines related to sex and bedtime behaviour. As the great *Mughals* ruled over their Indian empire from Delhi, this branch of medicinal science, relating to aphrodisiac applications, literally reached its royal heights. The *harem* was an extraordinary concept of the Mughal establishment, where a single man was supposed to satisfy the physical needs of a large number of women. Naturally, matters pertaining to the king's libido were discussed and worked out in great detail every night. The culture of keeping several wives became common practice for those who governed the territory. The *harem* was jealously guarded and no other male was allowed inside its precincts.

The King of Burma had 70 wives. He used a less toxic aconite, *Indian Atees* (*aconitum heterophyllum*), as an aphrodisiac. Multiple herbs and spices were used for the enhancement of sexual capacity in the Mughal period. Aphrodisiacs for men was divided into substances that increased excitability, those that strengthened the nerves and prevented premature ejaculations, and lastly substances that promoted the production of semen and fertility. An enlargement of the phallus was achieved by the application of pastes of poisonous insects; some of them were very painful, at times leading to blistering and ulceration. Such inflictions did not suit the temperaments of the Mughals, and were gradually replaced by the application of a paste made of spices. The male organ was hardened by massaging it with medicated oils of minerals like *arsenic trioxide*, and herbal oils containing the popular *Ashvagandha* or almond oil. Agents were also available to enhance vaginal contractility.

The dinner menu was important. Several exotic food preparations were served to enhance sexual desire. Bizarre preparations were described to achieve the desired effect and an inexhaustible supply of semen. Here are two typical recipes.

- Take a quantity of pork. Pound or grind it add mineral salt and the pepper. Make boluses and fry with clarified butter oil. Add meat juices of fowl that is enriched by the addition of perfumes, curd and fruit of pomegranate.

- Take some eggs of alligators and also some eggs of hen. Fry them in hot clarified butter oil. Mix them with *shastika* rice and fresh clarified butter. Make some cakes of the product. After taking the cakes, drink a glass of *Varuni* wine. Through the virtue of these cakes, one could approach women like stallion and discharge his seeds like an elephant.

Among the somewhat less exotic aphrodisiacs, milk boiled with the testes of he-goat was most commonly used. Later, for Hindu vegetarian pleasure-seekers, the testes of the he-goat was replaced by nuts such as almonds. In the Mughal royal house, the opium eating habit often began at a young age and was used as an aphrodisiac to postpone or delay orgasm. The Mughal nobility could not do without it and opium was secretly introduced into the *harem*, for the ladies in *purdah*.

Hindu society also rediscovered mechanisms from the ancient text of the *Kamasutra*, to keep sex vigour at a heightened level. *Hakims* and *Baids* were kept busy prescribing aphrodisiacal agents for the rich and noble, so much so that their interest in treating common disorders took a backseat. However, in spite of such a phenomenal development of the sex science in India between the 16th and 18th centuries, it remained beyond the reach of the common man. To this day, Indian society in general is too timid to talk about sex-related problems and diseases. It takes courage and special effort to overcome ingrained societal inhibitions and articulate sexual dysfunction. However, they still discreetly consume tonics and apply oils advertised in newspapers and on television channels, and drink milk boiled with nuts and dates for the wedding night.

LONGEVITY
One who knows; virtues
Of herbs & root is a man
Of water & fire is a spirit
Of prayer is a prophet
Of quick silver is a god
Elixirs, cosmetics, aphrodisiac, poisons were only too well known...

The ancient Indian science of *Rasayana* (alchemy), was founded in an attempt to convert mercury or gold into *amrita*. Later, this science fell into the dark of the mystic sciences. Notwithstanding such elements of occultism, partial practice of *Rasayana* is a constituent of today's naturopathy, used for detoxification of the body and its rejuvenation.

Ancient Ayurveda provided the basis for the *Baid*'s search for the fountain of youth and the elixir of immortality. Multiple herbs were described in Ayurveda for renewing youth. Of these, *Soma* was considered as the king of all herbs. It waxed and waned like the cycle of the moon. Its growth began in the lighted half of the month. On the first lunar day with light, only one leaf, and on the second, two leaves, grow. Thus, on the full moon day, the herb is adorned with 15 leaves. This, literature says, is the maximum number. The leaves fall off one by one during the dark half of the month, till on the day of the new moon, the herb is shorn of all its leaves. However, the *Soma* plant is supposedly invisible to the non-believer in its curative virtues and to those who are spiteful towards Brahmins.

A traditional operating procedure for attaining longevity runs on the following lines: after consuming the juices of rare herbs, the person lies down naked in a casket made of raw wood. Goat's milk is his only sustenance. This process continues for six months, at which stage, he becomes celestial in age, complexion, voice, shape, strength and lustre. Svoboda, in his book *Ayurveda: Life, Health and Longevity*, described another methodology: on an auspicious day, after the performance of various rituals, the person goes into a hut where neither light nor wind can enter; and remains there in peaceful meditation for four to six weeks while the rejuvenating substances do their work. During this period, his hair, teeth and nails all fall out and re-grow, and he sheds his skin and renews it. Some decades ago, Pandit Madan Mohan Malaviya, the founder of the Benaras Hindu University, was given such a treatment by a yogi who had lived for more than 160 years; but Pandit Malviya, who could not endure all the restrictions, emerged before completion of the full course of treatment and so derived only moderate benefits.

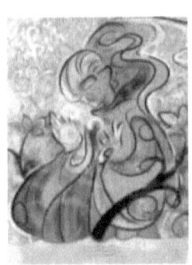

In Conclusion

The Indian nation is now served by a multiplicity of medicinal systems claiming to treat acute and chronic illnesses. Alternative medicines are freely advertised and sold across the country without proven scientific validity or any regulatory mechanism worth the name. The problem stares us in the face, yet the much-needed integration of various medical systems remains a distant dream. People are free to choose any modality of treatment as a matter of faith, and may even die as the price of that faith.

Fearsome diseases like tuberculosis, leprosy and malaria have been covered under systems of national surveillance since independence. Still, these diseases have never been wiped out, nor even controlled in a proper fashion in spite of massive efforts. Such afflictions are linked to a lack of resources that undermines healthcare in the world's developing nations. The network of available healthcare generally comprises overcrowded state hospitals and mushrooming nursing homes in cities and quacks in rural areas; apart from those district hospitals with few resources that spend most of their time chasing national targets for health. There are, of course, higher-end institutes with multiple sub-specialists where the war between disease and medicine goes on to keep people alive, but a tribal member rarely even reaches the age of fifty.

An overstressed national health system is unable to provide updated medical facilities in rural India. Modern medicine consisting of vaccinations, medication and surgery has failed to reach the people who need it the most. Qualified doctors simply dislike serving villages, and without them, reaching some 638,000 odd villages remains a herculean task. Nowhere is the gaping divide between the two Indias – the rural and urban India; or the educated and un-educated India – more pathetic from a basic humanitarian perspective, than in the field of medical care. Tropical medicine is not only about differential disease patterns in the tropics; it is more about the aspects of organisation, availability and delivery of the medical system in tropical countries.

The problems of economically challenged population; the growing burden of diseases and disabilities on limited resources; the harm done by ineffective, toxic and unsafe treatments; and on top of all that, lack of a people's safety net of affordable medical insurance, make survival difficult for the vast majority of citizens. The country surely deserves a better infrastructure for public health and an integrated medical system.

****

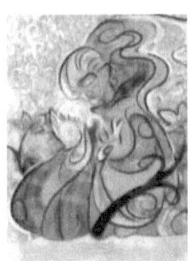

APPENDICES

APPENDIX 1

Incidence of Major Illness Perception Analysis in Chhattisgarh (CG) (Jan Rapats – Part III 2005)

	Factor	Percentage
1.	Polluted water	38.1
2.	Lack of hygiene	44.3
3.	Stale food	20.3
4.	Alcohol	38.3
5.	Illiteracy	2.6
6.	Pollution	2.8

Factors Responsible for Poor Health: Percentage of Village Reports Selected for Perception Analysis (2005)

	Disease	Incidence in CG
1.	Malaria	40.2
2.	Diarrhoea	53.9
3.	Leprosy	1.2
4.	Tuberculosis	1.96
5.	Skin disease	3.1
6.	Stomach-related ailments	21.5
7.	Headache	5.25
8.	Cholera	15.2
9.	Snakebite	14.1

Source: Chhattisgarh human development report; Govt of Chhattisgarh 2005; p.12

APPENDIX 2

Cause of illness among 100 admissions in army (1895 – 1900)

	European (British) Troop	Indian (Native) Troop
Intermittent Fever	22.6	38.3
Venereal Disease	31.2	4.6
Dysentery	5.9	2.3
Respiratory Disease	1.8	3.6

Mortality among 100 admissions in army (1895-1900)

European (British) troops	
Gastrointestinal Causes	Enteric Fever
	Hepatic Abscess
	Dysentery
All deaths related to gut illness	
Indian (native) troops	
Respiratory Causes	Pneumonia
	Tubercle of Lung
	Respiratory Disease
All deaths related to Respiratory illness	

Source: Imperial Gazetteer2 of India, Volume 1, p. 533.

APPENDIX 3

Major Killers during the British era

Cause of death	Years	Deaths in millions
Smallpox*	1871–1900	0.37
Plague*	1896–1903	2.1
Famine**	1875–1900	26

Source: *Imperial Gazetteer of India, Volume 1, 467
**Wikipedia

APPENDIX 4

Natural history of pulmonary tuberculosis:
Before the availability of effective anti-tubercular drugs in sanatoria

Tuberculosis	Total No. of Patients	No. of survivors at 5 years
Stage-1 (Early TB)	257	214 (83.3 per cent)
Stage-2 (Established TB)	324	207 (63.9 per cent)
Stage-3 (Advanced TB)	383	71 (18.5 per cent)

Source: Frimodt-Moller C. IMG 1931

APPENDIX 5

Number of snakebite-related deaths & number of snakes killed (1880-1881)

Year	No. of deaths due to snake bite	No. of Snakes Killed
1880	19060	212,776
1881	18610	254,968

Source: BMJ

APPENDIX 6

Number of epileptics in various lunatic asylums in British India

	Number of Epileptics	Per cent
United Province	23	7.03 per cent
Lahore	-	8.09 per cent
Central Province	17	5.55 per cent*
Assam	16	4.57 per cent
Madras	-	25 per cent*

Relative numbers of different Epileptics classified as Lunatics in the mental asylums (1898)

	Bengal	Madras	Punjab
Mania with Epilepsy	39	43	33
Melancholia with Epilepsy	4	–	–
Dementia with Epilepsy	3	1	4
TOTAL	46/1083 (4.24 %)	44/714 (6.16 %)	37/558 (6.63 %)

Source: The Indian Medical Gazette (1899)

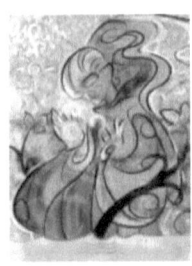

Glossary of Terms

Acetaminophen	Paracetamol
Acute Flaccid Paralysis	Floppy weakness of limbs of recent origin
Adenosine Deaminase	An enzyme that is involved in purine metabolism
Agharia	A caste belonging to some districts in Orissa and Chhattisgarh states in India. They claim to be of the Kshatriya caste in the Hindu class division.
Albuminuria	The presence of albumin in the urine
Amblyopia	Lazy eye
Amphotericin	An antifungal drug that is used to treat deep-seated fungal infections
Amyotrophic Lateral Sclerosis	A progressive loss of muscle bulk associated with flickering and twitching in the muscles
Anaemia	A reduction in the quantity of the oxygen carrying pigment haemoglobin
Anna	One-sixteenth of a rupee.
Apasmara	Sanskrit word for Epilepsy
Apoplexy	Stroke
Arteriole	A small branch of an artery leading into many smaller vessels.
Arthashastra	Ancient Indian treatise on state affairs, economic & foreign policy, by Kautilya
Arthrogryposis Multiplex Congenita	Multiple joint contractures from birth

Glossary of Terms

Asana	Different body positions adopted in the practice of Yoga
Ashtaavakra	A sage mentioned in Hindu scriptures
Ashvagandha (*Withania somnifera*)	Indian ginseng
Aspergilloma	Fungal granuloma caused by aspergillus invasion
Atees	An Indian aconite, non-poisonous plant of medicinal value.
Atharvaveda	Sacred Hindu text one of the four *Veda*s
Atonic Dyspepsia	Floppy stomach leading to decreased appetite
Bacillus	Any rod-shaped bacterium.
Badi Mata	Small pox
Baid	Term used in India to refer to a person or doctor practicing Ayurveda
Barbiturate	Drug used for sedation, with anaesthetic and antiepileptic properties
Basi	A fermented rice preparation
Bataasha	Sugar bubble
Bazaar	Native market
Begum	Noble lady
Bhangh	Preparation from the leaves and flowers (buds) of the female cannabis plant, smoked or consumed as a beverage in the Indian subcontinent
Brahmi	Small herb popular as a nerve tonic
Brahmins	Name used to designate one of the four castes in traditional Hindu society
Brain Fever Bird	The hawk-cuckoo.
Bronchitis	Inflammation of the bronchi
Calisayan	Bark of a tropical tree such as *cinchona*
Cantonment	Military area
Cardiazol (*Pentylenetrazol*)	Drug used to cause convulsion
Catatonia	A state in which a person becomes mute and adopts a bizarre, rigid posture

Glossary of Terms

Cerebral White Matter	Deeper brain tissue covered by grey matter
Cerebrospinal Meningitis	Inflammation of covering of the brain
Chai	A beverage made by brewing tea with a mixture of aromatic Indian spices, herbs, milk and sugar
Chamunda	The Hindu Divine Mother and one of the seven *Maatrika*s (mother goddesses)
Charak Puja	Folk festival of the southern belt of Bangladesh and West Bengal
Charas (Cannabis Sativa/ Cannabis Indica)	Resin of the cannabis plant
Chaulmoogra	Large tree in South East Asia; source of *chaulmoogra* and *hydnocarpus* oils
Chlorhexidine solution	Common ingredient in mouthwash
Chhota	Small
Chhoti mata	Chicken pox
Cicatrix	Scar
Cleft palate and lip	Gap in the lip and palate
Clonic	Spasm-like
Clostridium Tetani	Organism responsible for tetanus
Coatee	A short coat
Collagen	Repairing tissue
Convulsion	Seizure / Fit
Cooly	Porter
Cortico Venous Thrombosis	Stasis of blood in venous drainage of the brain
Cutaneous lentigines	Birth spots the size of lentil grains
Cutis Vertices Gyrate	Folded skin on scalp
Datura	Seeds of flowering plants belonging to the *Solanaceae* family
Dementia	Decline in memory
Demyelination	Loss of nerve covering
Dextropropoxyphene	Opiate analgesic
Dhobi	Indian washerman

Glossary of Terms

Dhobi-itch	Skin infection, usually ringworm
DIC (Disseminated Intravascular Coagulation)	Defective blood coagulation causing excessive bleeding (internal & external)
Dicyclomine Hydrochloride	Reduces spasm of smooth muscle
Dilantin	Brand name for phenytoin sodium
Dystonia	Abnormal muscle contraction leading to abnormal posture
Eclampsia	Convulsion/s associated with hypertension and albumin in urine during pregnancy
Encephalomyelitis	Inflammation of brain and spinal cord.
Endemic	Occurring frequently in a particular region or population
Enterovirus	Any virus that enters the body through the gastrointestinal tract
Fasciotomy	Cutting through a layer below the skin
Febrifuge	Powder form of cinchona bark (contains crude quinine)
Fibrosis	Scar with collagen fibres
Fluorosis	Fluoride toxicity
Forrard	Forward
Fundus Examination	Visual examination of inner eye and retina with ophthalmoscope
Gandhak	Sulphur / Sulphuric acid derivatives
Ganja	A term (of Sanskrit origin) for cannabis
General Paresis	Advanced state of neurosyphilis
Generalised Tonic-Clonic Seizure	Type of convulsion, characterised by stiffening of body fallowed by jerks
Ghotu	Bread made of *Lathyrus sativus* flour
Gingival hyperplasia/Gum hyperplasia	Overgrowth of gums
Gluteus Muscle	Thick muscle of buttocks
Glycosuria	Excreting glucose in urine
Grierson-Gopalan Syndrome	Burning feet syndrome
Gyri	Folds on surface of brain

Glossary of Terms

Haemeralopia	Day blindness
Haemolytic	Lysis of blood components
Hakgala Gardens	Botanical garden near Nuwara Eliya, in Sri Lanka
Hakim	Persian physician
Harem	Palace for female members of the family
Herpes Infection	Reactivation of dormant herpes virus
Hindu	Majority population indigenous to the Indian subcontinent
Hydnocarpus	Plants used to extract Chaulmoogras
Hydrocele	Enlarged scrotal sac due to accumulation of fluid
Hydrophobia	Aversion to water; a sign of rabies
Hyperaemia	Increased circulation
Hyperesthesia	Increased sensation of touch
Hyperpyrexia	Very high body temperature
Hypoxic	Lack of oxygen
Imbecile	Individual with moderate to severe mental retardation
Immunisation	Being vaccinated
Indian Medical Service (IMS)	Military medical services in India during British rule.
Infant mortality	Death of children below one year
Inoculation	Delivery inside the body
Insane	Mad
Insomnia	Lack of sleep
Interictal Psychosis	Madness between convulsive episodes
Intramuscular	Inside muscle
Jats	A traditional community of tillers and herders in north India and Pakistan
Kamasutra	Ancient Indian erotic literature
Kapha	In Ayurveda, *Kapha* is responsible for lubrication in the body

Glossary of Terms

Kautilya	Celebrated politician and minister of Emperor Chandragupta Maurya in Indian history; author of *Arthashastra*.
Konark	A small town in the Puri District in the state of Orissa, India, on the Bay of Bengal; known for its famous sun temple.
Krait	A genus of venomous snakes found in South and South-East Asia.
Krishna	A central figure of Hinduism; the 'Blessed Lord' to whom the telling of the Bhagavad Gita is traditionally attributed.
Kumbh	Mass Hindu pilgrimage in which devotees gather at the Ganges River at Prayag/Allahabad once in twelve years.
Kumbha	A full vase, pot, a jar or a pitcher.
Lathi	Stick, also refers to an Indian martial art based on cane fighting.
Lumbricus	Small muscles in hand.
Lunatic	Mad person.
Macrocytic anaemia	Anaemia with bigger red blood cell.
Madak	A blend of opium and tobacco used as a recreational drug in 17th and 18th century China, India
Mahamrityunjaya Mantra	Verse of the Rigveda invoking god Tryambaka to conquer death; another name for Rudra/Shiva.
Mahua	An Indian tropical tree found largely in the central and north Indian plains and forests. Flowers are fermented for preparation of wine.
Majum	A strong preparation of cannabis and opium.
Mal de mer	French term for seasickness.
Malignant Anaemia	Chronic, progressive anaemia in older adults
Mallotus Philippensis	Plant with wormicidal properties

Glossary of Terms

Malta	Type of fever
Mania	Madness
Marhi	A shanty town of roadside restaurants located on the Manali-Leh highway in Himachal Pradesh, India
Masseter Muscle	Jaw muscle responsible for clenching
Mastak	Sanskrit word for brain
Melancholia	Psychiatric depression/disturbances
Metabolic	Relating to the chemical process within a living body
Microcephalic Head	Small-sized head
Morvan's Fibrillary Chorea	Syndrome of twitching and tremors due to malignant /non–malignant conditions
Mucous Colitis	Bowel dysfunction related to the passage of mucous in stool
Mughals	Timurid invaders and rulers of India
Multicystic Encephalomalacia	Severe hypoxic brain damage in infants
Multiple Sclerosis	Demyelinating disease
Murchha	Fainting fit; senseless condition
Mycobacterium	Organism responsible for TB
Mycotic	Fungal
Neuralgia	Neuropathic pain
Neuraxis	Craniospinal axis
Neuropathic Pain	Pain originating in neural structure (usually peripheral)
Nyctalopia	Night blindness
Opioid	Opium-related
Optic disk	Part of retina
Osteogenesis	Imperfect ossification; impure bone with glass-like fragility
Pagri	Turban
Palanquin	A couch carried by four men (*Kahar* / bearers), with four others as reserves
Pantothenate	Vitamin B5
Parkinsonism	Disease with excessive tremors

Glossary of Terms

Parotitis	Inflammation of parotid salivary glands
Paroxysms	Episodic/ intermittent/ sharp recurrence of symptoms
Phuljharia/ Raigarhia/Ratanpuria	Division of the Agharia caste, named on geographical distribution
Pilocarpine	Acetylcholine-like drugs
Pitta	In Ayurveda, *pitta* is associated with fire or heat and responsible for metabolism
Polio	A viral disease that can affect nerves and lead to partial or full paralysis
Poliomyelitis	A disease leading to paralysis of limbs, usually in childhood
Polioviruses	Virus causing poliomyelitis
Polyneuritis Cranialis	Multiple cranial neuropathies
Posterior Fossa	Hind part of the brain cavity
Prallethrin	Compound used to kill mosquitos
Prophylaxis	Prevention
Propoxyphene Napsylate	Painkiller
Psychosomatic Disorder	Involving both the mind and body
Puerperal Convulsions	Convulsions related to childbirth
Putamen	Part of the lenticular nucleus (Basal ganglionic complex)
Putaminal Necrosis	Destruction of putamen
Pyrexial Therapy	Disease treated with fever like mania
Quinine Hypobromide	A quinine salt
Rabies Vaccine	Immunisation against rabies virus
Rasayana	Alchemy
Refractory Epileptics	Epilepsy not adequately controlled with drugs
Rhinosporidiosis	A fungal infection of the mucous membranes of the nose, larynx and eyes, caused by fungus
Rigveda	The oldest of the four sacred texts of Hinduism, known as the *Vedas*

Glossary of Terms

Rudra/Shiva	The destroyer or transformer god of the Hindu Trinity
Sadhu	Indian holy man
Sannipat	A disorder of the bodily humours
Saptamatrika	Seven Mothers – a group of Hindu Mother-Goddesses who are always depicted together: *Brahmani, Vaishnavi, Maheshwari, Indrani, Kaumari, Varahi* and *Chamunda/Narasimhi*
Saree	A length of unstitched cloth of 4-9 yards, worn by women in India
Schizophrenia	Severe mental disorder, characterised by disintegration of personality
Sciatic Nerve	Major nerve of the leg, with the largest diameter, from the lumbar region down
Seetla (Sitala)	A Hindu goddess widely worshipped as the pox-goddess
Seizures	Convulsions/fits
Sendri Mata	Measles
Sensory Dermatomes	Areas of skin supplied by a single nerve root for sensation
Shah Jahan	The Mughal Emperor from 1628 -1658. The name 'Shah Jahan' means 'King of the World' in Persian
Shah Shuja	Second son of the Mughal Emperor Shah Jahan and Mumtaz Mahal
Sham Mirth	False smile
Sharab	Wine or other alcoholic drinks
Shastika	Variety of rice considered cool and tasty and a rectifier of the imbalance of basic elements in the body
Shavites	Followers of Shiva
Shirodhara	A form of Ayurveda that involves gently pouring liquids over the forehead (the 'third eye')
Sickle Cell Carriers/ Sickle Cell Trait	Defective gene inherited from a parent

Glossary of Terms

Siddha	'One who is accomplished'; refers to perfected masters
Snake Stone	A stone made of herbal ashes, bone and other ingredients with marked hygroscopic properties. It is used to absorb poison from snakebite sites
Spasmo-Proxyvon	Branded painkiller in India
Stroke	Sudden attack of weakness affecting one side of the body
Stupes	Any piece of material or wad of cotton wool, soaked in hot water and medicine
Suppurative Parotitis	Formation of pus in the parotid gland.
Surya	Sun
Sushruta	Ancient Indian surgeon and author of the *Sushruta Samhita*, in which he describes over 300 surgical procedures, 120 surgical instruments, and classifies human surgery into 8 categories
Sutak	The impure period after birth and death and a solar or lunar eclipse
Taenia	A flat ribbon-like anatomical structure or genus of a large tapeworm
Tapti	One of the major rivers of peninsular India with a length of about 724 kms
Tezaab	Sulphuric acid
Tinea	Ringworm
Tissue Necrosis	Death or destruction of groups of cells
Tonhi	Term for a witch, in Chhattisgarh
Topee	Lightweight hat worn in the tropcs for protection from the sun
Toxaemia	Blood contamination caused by toxins formed by the growth of bacteria
Toxic Encephalopathy	Toxin affecting brain sensorium
Trans-Allethrin	A compound to kill mosquitos
Treponema Pallidum	A genus of spirochaete bacteria responsible for syphilis

Glossary of Terms

Trismus	Spasm of the jaw muscles which clamps the jaw shut
Tubercle	Granuloma of tuberculosis
Tunica Vaginalis	Layer of testis
Typhus	Spotted fever
Unnao	The headquarters of Unnao district, Uttar Pradesh, India, located between Kanpur and Lucknow
Vaccinations	Means of producing immunity to a disease through a vaccine
Varices	Varicose/dilated veins
Varuna	God of the sky, water and ocean
Varuni	An ancient wine
Vata	In Ayurveda, *vata* refers to the movement of *Vayu* (air), inside the body
Vayu	Lord of the winds
Vedic	A large body of texts composed in Vedic Sanskrit, from ancient India
Vertebra (plural: *Vertebrae*)	One of 33 bones in the spine
Voriconazole	Antifungal drug
Yajurveda	The third of the four ancient texts of Hinduism, the *Vedas*
Yogi	Hindu ascetic.
Yunani	Arabic system of medicine

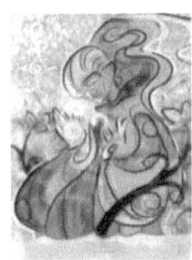

REFERENCES

INTRODUCTION
1. Cayley H. *Notes on Ladakh in 1867*; Indian Medical Gazette, Jan. 1868; p. 3
2. Roy SB, Sen SK. *Scientific research papers by native Bengali authors during the nineteenth century*; Current Science, Vol. 99, No. 12, December 2010; 1849-1857
3. Rao MS. *The history of medicine in India and Burma; A paper read at the Symposium on The History of Medicine in the Commonwealth*, organized by the faculty of the History of Medicine and Pharmacy, and held at the Royal College of Physicians of London, September, 1936; pp. 52-61
4. *Chhattisgarh human development report*; Government of Chhattisgarh, 2005; pp. 124-128
5. *London letters. Some Indian Friends and Acquaintances*; Indian Medical Gazette, December 1904; p. 164
6. Soni S. *India's Glorious Scientific Tradition*; Ocean Paperbacks, 2009; p. 178

CHAPTER 1 MEDICINE
7. *Mahatma Gandhi and Ayurveda* — Indian Medical Record, August 1925; Indian Medical Gazette, December 1925; pp. 592-593
8. Civil Surgeon (anonymous). *Hint from a Hakeem*; Indian Medical Gazette, May 1868; p. 105
9. Lockwood KP. *Beast and Man in India*, Macmillan and co., 1904; p. 24
10. *Vaidyak Sarangdhar Bhashatika*; July 1889
11. Rangarajan LN. *Kautilya the Arthashastra*; Penguin books, 1992; p. 105
12. Habib I. *Medieval India The study of a civilization*; National Book Trust, India, 2008, pp. 22-23 & 76
13. Wills CJ. *Medicine in Persia*, BMJ, 1879; pp. 623-624
14. Patel V, Kirkwood B, Weiss H, Pednekar S, Fernandes J, Pereira B, Upadhye M, Mabey D. *Chronic Fatigue in developing countries. Population-based survey of women in India*; Vol. 330, May 2005; p. 1190
15. Culpin M. *An Examination of Tropical Neurasthenia; Section of Tropical Diseases and Parasitology*, Proceedings of the Royal Society of Medicine; 1933; pp. 911-922

16. *Neurasthenia among Europeans in India*; BMJ, March 1914; p. 727
17. Sleeman. *Rambles and Recollections*, 1833
18. Allen C. *Plain tales from The Raj*; Abacus, 1994; p. 209

CHAPTER 2 QUACKS, ILLNESS & SUPPORT

19. *Chhattisgarh human development report*; Government of Chhattisgarh, 2005; pp. 124,128
20. *A Plea for Hakeems*; Indian Medical Gazette, April 1968; p. 87
21. Justitia. *A Protest against Quackery of all kinds to the editor of the 'Hindu Patriot'*; Indian Medical Gazette, July 1868; pp. 162-163
22. Harris JG. *Tales of the first firangis*: Hindustan Times weekly magazine, December 2011
23. *Indigenous Medical Systems of India*; BMJ, February 1892; p. 345
24. Cayley H. *Notes on Ladakh in 1867*; Indian Medical Gazette, Jan 1868; p. 3
25. Sen SN. *Indian travels of Jean De Thevenot 1666-1667 and Gemelli Careri 1695-1696*; National archives of India, Asian educational services, 1949
26. Oudhia P. *Traditional Medicinal Knowledge about common herbs, insects and mites used in treatment of Lakwa (Paralysis) in Chhattisgarh, India.* http://botanical.com/site/column_poudhia/102_mirgi.html

CHAPTER 3 EPIDEMICS, INFECTION & PREVENTION

27. *Indian Pilgrims and Mecca*; Indian Medical Gazette, November 1893; 381
28. Chernin E, Haffkine RD. Ross Defends Haffkine: *The Aftermath of the Vaccine-Associated Mulkowal Disaster of 1902*; Journal of the history of medicine and allied sciences, Inc., 1991, SSN 0022-5045 Volume 46; pp. 201-218
29. *Haffkine's Antiplague Prophylactic*; BMJ, February 1907; p. 285
30. Nalin DR. *The Cover Art of the 15 June, 2004 Issue*; December 2004; pp. 1741-1742
31. Ronald R. *The Inoculation Accident at Mulkowal*; Nature, Volume 75, 1951; pp. 486-487
32. Liston WG. *The Milroy Lectures, 1924, on the Plague; The Epidemiology of Plague*; BMJ, June 1924; p. 997
33. Hamilton G. *Medical notes in Parliament*; BMJ, June 1903; p. 1335
34. *Scientific Investigation of Epidemic and Endemic Diseases*; BMJ, February 1914; p. 314
35. Dennys GWP. *Destruction of Rats as a means for the prevention of Plague*; Indian Medical Gazette, January 1918; p. 1
36. Sleeman. *Rambles and Recollections*; 1833
37. Bhagwat AK. Pradhan GP. Lokmanya Tilak: *A Biography Storm and stress*; Jaico, 2008; pp. 166-215

38. Napier: *The principal and practice of tropical medicine*, 1946, p. 372
39. Nelson AE. *Central Provinces district gazetteers*: Raipur District

CHAPTER 4 THE AUTUMNAL SCOURGE: MALARIA

40. Ewart J. *Cinchona Cultivation in British Sikkim*; Indian Medical Gazette, August 1868; pp. 176-179, 199-200
41. Meyer WS. *The Imperial gazetteer of India*, 1908-1931; Oxford, Clarendon Press, Volume 21; p. 50
42. Meyer WS. *The Imperial gazetteer of India*, Oxford, Clarendon Press, 1908-1931; Volume 3; pp. 66-69
43. *The Quinine Fraud*; Indian Medical Gazette, October 1939; p. 623
44. *The Quest for Quinine*; Indian Medical Gazette, July 1918; p. 261
45. *Cinchona supplies in India*; Indian Medical Gazette, June 1938; p. 353
46. Anderson FT. *The Introduction of cinchona trees into India*; BMJ, February 1916; p. 293

CHAPTER 5 AFFLICTIONS ON THE WANE – SYPHILIS & YAWS

47. Wise. *General Paralysis of the insane*; Indian Medical Gazette; April 1869, p. 75
48. Berkeley-Hill. *A Wassermann survey of the inmates of the Ranchi European Lunatic Asylum*; Indian Medical Gazette, March 1921; pp. 89-90
49. Taylor W, Richardson J. *Health of the troops in India*; BMJ, March 1897; p. 810
50. Wyman AG. *The decrease of venereal disease in the Indian Army*; BMJ; January 1900, p. 48
51. *Syphilisation*; Indian Medical Gazette, May 1868; p. 112.
52. *Lock Hospitals in Calcutta*; Indian Medical Gazette, December 1868; p. 281
53. Boeck. *Syphilisation as a means of curing constitutional syphilis*; BMJ, April 1865.
54. Castellani AI, Chalmers AJ. *A manual of tropical medicine*; Annual of tropical medicine 31, 1919
55. *Yaws; Tropical medical and Hygiene*; BMJ; July 1917, p. 105
56. Kipling R. *Something of myself*; September 1991
57. *Yaws; Elimination in India a step towards Eradication* Government of India, World Health Organization, September 2006
58. *Insanity in India*; Indian Medical Gazette, October 1899; p. 373

CHAPTER 6 THE PERCEIVED CURSE: LEPROSY

59. *The ancient and leprosy*; Indian Medical Gazette, November 1893; pp. 380-1
60. Meyer WS, *The Imperial Gazetteer of India*; Oxford, Clarendon Press, 1908-1931; Volume 7; p. 104

61. Meyer WS, *The Imperial Gazetteer of India*, Oxford, Clarendon Press, 1908-1931; Volume 8; p. 123
62. Meyer WS, *The Imperial Gazetteer of India*, Oxford, Clarendon Press, 1908-1931; Volume 17; p. 149
63. Meyer WS, *The Imperial Gazetteer of India*, Oxford, Clarendon Press, 1908-1931; Volume 23; p. 252
64. Meyer WS, *The Imperial Gazetteer of India*, Oxford, Clarendon Press, 1908-1931; Volume 23; p. 392
65. Prascandola J. *Chaulmoogra Oil and the Treatment of Leprosy*;
    www.lhnbc.nlm.nih.gov/lhc/docs/published/.../pub2003048.pdf
66. *Leprosy in India*; BMJ, April 1893; p. 806
67. *Medical Missionaries in India*; Indian Medical Gazette, February 1904; p. 69
68. Hutchinson Sir J. *Obituary*; BMJ, June 1913; p. 1398
69. Lang MC. *Treatment of Leprosy*; BMJ, September 1927
70. Rogers L. *Tuberculosis incidence and climate in India*; BMJ, February 1925; p. 256
71. Magic and Medicine of Plants, Reader's Digest, 1986, p. 366

CHAPTER 7 LIVING IN HOPE: TUBERCULOSIS
72. Frimodt-Moller C. *An investigation of after histories of sanatorium patients in India*; Indian Medical Gazette, September 1931; pp. 484-487
73. *Alberuni's India*, Translated by Sachau EC; WW Norton & Company. INC. 1971; pp. 140-141
74. Colditz GA, Brewer TF, Berkley CS, et al. *Efficacy of BCG vaccine in the prevention of tuberculosis*; JAMA, 1994, pp. 271; 698-702
75. Rogers L. *Tuberculosis incidence and Climate in India: Rainfall and Winds*; BMJ; February 1925; p. 256
76. Lankester A. *Tuberculosis in India: Its prevalence, causation & prevention*; Butterworth & Co. (India), 1920; pp. 12-13

CHAPTER 8 WORMS IN THE GUT & BRAIN: NEUROCYSTICERCOSIS
77. Reddy DJ. *A case of cysticercosis*: Indian Medical Gazette, January 1951; pp. 14-15
78. Armstrong H. *A case of Cysticercus Cellulosae of the brain*; Indian Medical Gazette, August 1888; p. 252
79. Dave CJ. *Generalized Cysticercosis Cellulose*; Indian Medical Gazette, March 1950; pp. 92-94
80. Luving J. *Note on Embelia Ribes as a remedy for Tapeworm*; Indian Medical Gazette, May 1869; p. 92
81. McRobert G.R. *Somatic Taeniasis (Solium Cysticercosis)*; Indian Medical Gazette, September 1944; pp. 399-400

82. Prakash V, Mehrotra BN. *Anthelmintic Plants in Traditional Remedies in India*, Indian Journal of History of Science, 22(4): March 1987; pp. 332-340
83. Fleming J. *Remarks on Cyst- Infected Meat at Meean Meer, its Nature and Prevention*; Indian Medical Gazette, June 1869; pp. 114-115
84. Waring EJ. *Remarks on the uses of the bazaar medicines and common medical plants of India*, 1883
85. *Magic and Medicine of Plants*; Reader's Digest, 1986; p. 362

CHAPTER 9 FUNGUS

86. Elliston G. *Meetings of branches and divisions*; BMJ, April 1909; p. 156
87. McCarrison R. *India and Medical Progress*; BMJ, July 1917; p. 109
88. Mosny E. *Infectious diseases of the skin and Mucosa*; BMJ, Sept. 1911; p. 690
89. Rangarajan LN. *Kautilya: the Arthashastra*; Penguin books, 1992; p. 215
90. Allen C. *Plain tales from The Raj*; Abacus, 1994; p. 150
91. Castellani AI Chalmers AJ. *A manual of tropical medicine*; 31st Annual of tropical medicine; 1919.
92. Napier: *The principal and practice of tropical medicine*; 1946; p. 578
93. Russell RV. *The Tribes and Castes of the Central Provinces of India – Dhobi*; Volume II, p. 519

CHAPTER 10 STIFF SPINE & TETANUS

94. *The office of public vaccinator, Correspondence*; BMJ, February 1907; p. 344.
95. Inglis J. *Case of Traumatic Tetanus-Exhibition of the Extract of Indian Hemp (Cannabis Indica)-Death-Autopsy*; The provincial medical and surgical journal, 1845; pp. 112-114.
96. *Against Tetanus*; BMJ; January 1943; p. 76
97. O'Shaughnessy WB. *On the preparations of the Indian Hemp, or Gunjah*; London, Saturday, February 1843; pp. 363-369

CHAPTER 11 HEAT, DUST & MENINGITIS

98. Russell AJH. *Cerebrospinal Meningitis in India*; The Indian Medical Journal, January 1936; Vol XXX No.1; p. 1211
99. Buchanan WJ. *A Contribution to the Aetiology of Epidemic Cerebrospinal Meningitis.* J of Hyg (London), April 1901, 1(2); pp. 214–227
100. Good J. *A case of Paralysis Agitans, 'Parkinson's Palsy' with a note on its causation*; Indian Medical Gazette; February 1904; p. 60
101. Robb AG. *Encephalitis Lethargica; medical press and circular*, March 4, 1925; p. 173. Indian Medical Gazette, 1925; pp. 287-288
102. Dhunjibhoy JE. *Encephalitis Lethargica—A brief Description of the disease, with short notes on the post-encephalitic lethargic cases treated at the Ranchi Indian Mental Hospital*, Indian Medical Gazette; July 1929; pp. 362-363.

103. Sanders. *Cerebrospinal Fever*; Indian Medical Gazette, May 1886; p. 146

104. Stott H. *The use of Stramonium for the rigidity and drowsiness following encephalitis lethargica*, November 1935; p. 620

105. Ghosh PK. *Clinical Memoranda, Cerebral Malaria or Encephalitis Lethargica*; BMJ, 1935; p. 162

106. Barry C. *Notes on A case of Puerperal Eclampsia Treated by Hypodermic Injection of Morphia*; Indian Medical Gazette, February 1904; p. 60

107. Achard C. *The Differential Diagnosis of Encephalitis Lethargica*; Indian Medical Gazette, November 1921; p. 432

108. *Begums Thugs & Englishmen*; Journals of Fanny Parks; Penguin Books, 2003; p. 64

CHAPTER 12 THE ANGRY GODDESS: SKIN-SPOTS

109. Harvey R. *The Peking Hospital*; Indian Medical Gazette, May 1869; p. 93.

110. Friedman M, Friedman GW. *Medicines' 10 greatest discoveries: Edward Jenner and Vaccination*; University Press, 2005; pp. 65-93

111. Habib I. *Medieval India The study of a civilization*; National Book Trust, India, 2008; p. 201

112. Soni S. *India's Glorious Scientific Tradition*; Ocean Paperbacks, 2009; pp. 184-185

113. Parkes F. *Wanderings of pilgrim in search of the picturesque*, 1850

114. Wills CJ. *Medicine in Persia*, BMJ, 1879; pp. 623-624

CHAPTER 13 DOGBITE & RABIES

115. Ghose NT. *A case of hydrophobia cured by subcutaneous injection of hydrochlorate of pilocarpine*; Indian Medical Gazette, November 1891; p 341

116. *Letter to French academy*—M. Raman de la Sagra. *Progress of the medical and collateral sciences*; Indian Medical Gazette, November 1868; p. 262

117. Barnes JJ. *A case of hydrophobia successfully treated by salivation*; Indian Medical Gazette, May 1868; p. 106

118. *Scientific Investigation of Epidemic and Endemic Diseases*; BMJ, February 1914; p. 314

119. Cornwall JB. *The Ayurvedic Treatment of Rabies*; Indian Medical Gazette, August 1925; p. 76

120. *Ophidian Inoculation Progress of Medical and Collateral Sciences*; Indian Medical Gazette, November 1868; p. 263

121. McKendrick, FC. *The Pasteur Institute of India*; Indian Medical Gazette, June 1918; p. 361

122. Cormack HS. *Double Papilloedema Following Antirabic Inoculation: Recovery*; Indian Medical Gazette, August 1933; p. 459

123. Allen C. *Plain tales from The Raj*; Abacus, 1994; p. 29

CHAPTER 14 SNAKEBITE

124. *Original Communications experiments on the action of snake poison and its antidote*; Indian Medical Gazette, January 1869
125. Moors WJ. *A case of Snakebite*, Indian Medical Gazette; May 1868; pp 103-5
126. Mookerjee IB. *A case of Snakebite, cured by stimulants*, Indian Medical Gazette; June 1868; p. 132
127. *Experiments on the action of snake poison and its antidote* conducted at Gwalior Residency, in the presence of Colonel C.L. Showers, Officiating Political Agent; and Dr. J. Macbeth, Superintending Staff Surgeon of Morar. Indian Medical Gazette, 1869; pp. 1-3
128. *Ophidian Inoculation progress of medical and collateral sciences*; Indian Medical Gazette, November 1868; p. 263
129. Oudhia, P. *Common rice weeds used for first aid by Chhattisgarh farmers*. Agri. Sci. Digest. 21, 2001 (4); pp. 273-274
130. *Herbs and herbal constituents active against snake bite*; Indian Medical Gazette, September 2010; pp. 865-878
131. Elliot RH. *Treatment of Epilepsy by Snake Venom*; BMJ, December 1934; p. 1073
132. Rogers L. *Permanganate Treatment of Snake-Bite*; BMJ, August 1913; p. 345
133. Nicholson E. *Statistics of Deaths from Snakebite*; BMJ, September 1883; p 44
134. *Snakes and Predaceous Animals in India*; BMJ, December 1893; p. 1286
135. *Nova et Vetera*; BMJ, February 1904; p. 438
136. Travers B. *On the Arsenical Treatment of cases of Snakebite*; BMJ, Sept 1812
137. *Correspondence*; BMJ, August 1912; p. 457
138. Brunton TL. *Snake Venom and Its Antidotes*, Indian Medical Gazette; January 1891: London
139. EHA; *The Tribes on my Frontier*, 1914; Penguin-Viking 2007, *hypodermatikosyringophori*, p. 154
140. Nevile P. *Sahib's India Vignettes from the Raj*; Penguin Books, 2010; pp. 168-179
141. Oudhia P. *Traditional Medicinal Knowledge about common herbs used against venomous creatures snakes and scorpions in Chhattisgarh (India)* http://botanical.com/site/column_poudhia/02_venomous_creatures.html

CHAPTER 15 DEFORMITY

142. Lodge PC. *Microcephaly: A report on 'The Shah Dullah's Mice'*, Indian Medical Gazette; June 1928; pp. 297-301
143. Sullivan R. *Deformity — A modern western prejudice with ancient origins*; Proc Coll Physicians Edinh, 2001; pp. 31, 262-266
144. Mateen FJ, Boes CJ. *'Pinheads': The exhibition of neurologic disorders at 'The Greatest Show on Earth'*; Neurology; pp. 1-5

145. Williams GP, Leavitt L. Essay: *How Pan got his tail: The fusion of medicine, art, and myth*; Neurology, 2004, 62; pp. 519-522

146. *Human Oddities and Freaks*; BMJ, January 1935; p. 167

147. Ovington J. *A Voyage to Surat: The Faquirs near Surat*, 1696; pp. 361-67

148. Fryer J. *A New Account of East-India and Persia: A Description of Surat*, 1698; pp. 95, 102-103

149. EHA; *The Tribes on my Frontier*, 1914; Penguin-Viking 2007, hypodermatikosyringophori, p. 149

150. . Parkes F. *Wanderings of pilgrim in search of the picturesque; Residence at Cawnpore*, 1850

CHAPTER 16 HYDROCELE TAPPING

151. Gray Sr. GBD. *The injection treatment of Hydrocele*; BMJ, April 1930; p. 649.

152. Nicolson JW. *Treatment of Hydrocele by injection*; BMJ, August 1947; p. 188.

153. Rhind JA. *The Injection Treatment of Hydroceles and Spermatoceles*; BMJ, September 1951; p. 712

154. Vasavada DM. *Injection Treatment of Hydrocele*; Indian Medical Gazette, October 1931; p. 597

155. Castellani AI, Chalmers AJ. *A manual of tropical medicine*; 31st Annual of tropical medicine, 1919

CHAPTER 17 THE NERVE-TRAPPING INJECTION

156. Turner GG. *Site for Intramuscular Injection—Correspondence*; BMJ, July 1944; p. 56.

157. Biggam AG. *Damage of the Sciatic Nerve from Intramuscular Administration of Quinine*; BMJ, June 1930; p. 1171

CHAPTER 18 MEDICAL GEOLOGY: MANGANESE TOXICITY

158. Wadia NH. *Toxic effects of heavy metals in nervous system*. Neurology India, 1964; pp. 12, 29-41

159. Niyogi TP. Indian J. Indust, Medicine, 3, 1958; p.3.

160. *Manganese poisoning enquiry committee*, Ministry of Labour and Employment Government of India, 1960.

161. State Environment Report India, 2009

CHAPTER 19 SUN, MOON & WEATHER

162. Chatterjee SC. *The effect of lunar influence on Disease*; Indian Medical Gazette, June 1880; pp. 154-155

163. Logg RD. *Case of hemiplegia occurring after cold and damp, successfully treated by strychnia and galvanism*; Indian Medical Gazette, September 1868; p. 207

164. Faquhar T. *Apoplexy*; Indian Medical Gazette, July 1869; pp. 134-135
165. Waller WK. *Heat Apoplexy*; Indian Medical Gazette, July 1869; p. 132
166. Castellani AI, Chalmers AJ. *A manual of tropical medicine*; 31st Annual of tropical medicine, 1919
167. Moore WJ. *On Lunar Influence over Malarious fevers*; Indian MedicaGazette, June 1869; pp. 112-113
168. Moore WJ. *Maladies attributed to Lunar Influence,* Indian Medical Gazette; September 1800; p. 181
169. Johnson G. *The pathology and Treatment of Sun-Stroke*; BMJ, August 1868; p. 102
170. Finny CM. *Sunstroke or Heatstroke*; Indian Medical Gazette, October 1918; p. 361
171. Balfour F. Cupar; *A collection on treatises on the effects of sol- lunar influence on fevers with an improved method of curing them*, 1815
172. Nayar PK, Martin JR. Penguin books, 2009; p. 3

CHAPTER 20 DESPERATE SYMPTOMS CALL FOR DESPERATE REMEDIES: HEADACHE

173. Elmslir WJ. *Stray Notes on Chloroform*, Indian Medical Gazette; January 1868; p.5
174. Nunan W. *Mental Suggestion in Everyday Life*; Indian Medical Gazette, February 1934; p. 68
175. Sutherland WD. *Charaka Samhita*- Translated into English Published by Avinash Chandra Kaviratna, Calcutta page 186; Indian Medical Gazette, February 1919; pp. 41-50
176. Parkes F. *Wanderings of pilgrim in search of the picturesque*, p. 1850.
177. Nunan W. *Migraine and Suggestion*; Indian Medical Gazette, March 1928, pp. 169-171

CHAPTER 21 EPILEPTICS IN LUNATIC ASYLUMS & DRUGS TO TREAT EPILEPSY

178. Firth RH. *Epileptic Insanity*; Indian Medical Gazette, April 1886; pp 110-111
179. *Notes on current topics*; Indian Medical Gazette, May 1905, p. 187
180. Meyer WS, *The Imperial gazetteer of India*, Oxford, Clarendon Press, 1908-1931; Volume 4; pp. 465-466
181. Meyer WS. *The Imperial gazetteer of India*, Oxford, Clarendon Press, 1908-1931; Volume 24; p. 255
182. Meyer WS. *The Imperial gazetteer of India*, Oxford, Clarendon Press, 1908-1931; Volume 20; p. 375
183. Meyer WS. *The Imperial gazetteer of India*, Oxford, Clarendon Press, 1908-1931; Volume 10; p. 97

184. Meyer WS. *The Imperial gazetteer of India*, Oxford, Clarendon Press, 1908-1931; Volume 6; p. 106

185. Meyer WS. *The Imperial gazetteer of India*, Oxford, Clarendon Press, 1908-1931; Volume 16; p. 347

186. Staple PH, Reed MJ, Mashimo PA, Sedransk N, Umemoto T. *Diphenylhydantoin Gingival Hyperplasia in Macaca arctoides: Prevention by Inhibition of Dental Plaque Deposition*; Periodontol J.; Volume 49, Number 06, June 1978, p. 310

187. Edward JW. *Remarks on the uses of some of the Bazaar Medicines and common medical plants of India*. J.A. Churchill, 1897

188. Sharma S, Dasroy SKN. *Images in clinical medicine. Gingival hyperplasia induced by phenytoin*; Engl. J. Med. 2000

189. Elliot RH. *Treatment of Epilepsy by Snake Venom*; BMJ, December 1934; p. 1073

190. Prem Kishore, Padhi MM. *Common healing herbs*; Central Council for Research in Ayurveda & Siddha; Department of ISM & H, Ministry of Health and Family Welfare (Govt. of India) New Delhi, 2005

191. O'Shaughnessy WB. *On the preparations of the Indian Hemp, or Gunjah*; London, February 1843; pp. 363-369

192. Oudhia P. *Traditional Medicinal Knowledge about common herbs, insects and soils used in treatment of Mirgi (Epilepsy) in Chhattisgarh, India*; http://botanical.com/site/column_poudhia/93_mirgi.html

193. Oudhia P. *Bhang (Cannabis sativa) as medicinal herb in Chhattisgarh, India*; http://botanical.com/site/column_poudhia/articles/440_bhang.html

CHAPTER 22 SEIZURES OF DIFFERENT KIND

194. Taylor M. *Convulsion Therapy in Schizophrenia*; Indian Medical Gazette, October 1938; pp. 596-600

195. Finiefs LA. *Induced Epileptiform Attacks as a Treatment of Schizophrenia*; Indian Medical Gazette; January 1938, p. 52

196. McCabe DA. *Puerperal convulsions*; Indian Medical Gazette, August 1905; pp. 300-302

197. Barry C. *Notes on a case of Puerperal Eclampsia treated by Hypodermic injection of Morphia*; Indian Medical Gazette, February 1904; pp. 60-61

198. Balfour MI. *Obstetrics in India*; BMJ, December 1934; p. 1125

199. Taylor GF Chhuttani PN. *Nutritional Macrocytic Anaemia & the Animal Protein of Diet*; BMJ, June 1945; p. 800

200. Sippe GR. *Autolysed yeast in the treatment of Nutritional Macrocytic Anaemia*; BMJ, May 1944; p. 656

201. Smallwood WC. *The Anaemia of Pregnancy*; BMJ; London: September 1936

CHAPTER 23 CHILDREN & GENES

202. Sickle Cell Anaemia: *A Race specific Disease*; Indian Medical Gazette, April 1948; p. 200
203. Kar BC. *Sickle Cell Disease in India*; JAPI, 1991, Vol 39, No. 12; pp. 954-959.
204. *The Sickle- Cell Trait*; BMJ; February 1952, p. 426
205. Hoyte FC. *Obituary*; BMJ; August 1958, p. 332
206. Lehmann H. *Obituary*; BMJ; Volume 291, July 1985
207. Yasmeen K, et al. *International Journal of Applied Biology and Pharmaceutical Technology*; p. 718
208. Naik V. *Agharia Kshatriya*; Vikas 2007, p. 76

CHAPTER 24 THE DEFICIENT DIET

209. *Lathyrism in the central provinces*; Indian Medical Gazette, Dec. 1904; p.461
210. Gerrard PN. *Burning foot or Erythromelalgia Tropica*; Indian Medical Gazette, December 1904; p. 466
211. Ludolph AC, Hugon J, Dwivedi MP, Schaumburg HH, Spencer PS. *Studies on the Aetiology and Pathogenesis of Motor Neuron Diseases*; Brain, 1987; pp. 110, 149-165
212. Lambein F, Kuo KH. *Prevention of neurolathyrism during drought*; The Lancet; Volume 363, February 2004; p. 657
213. Dwivedi MP, Mishra SS. *Recent outbreak of Lathyrism and experience with propagation of detoxified L. Sativus*. Proc Nutr Soc India 1974; pp113: 345-76
214. *Advertisement*. Supplement to the Indian Medical Gazette No. 2, Vol. XX. *The Burroughs Beef and Iron Wine*; Indian Medical Gazette, 1867
215. Napier. *The principal and practice of tropical medicine*; 1946; p. 759
216. Sleeman. *Rambles and Recollections*; 1833
217. Edward JW. *Remarks on the uses of some of the Bazaar Medicines and common medical plants of India*. J.A. Churchill, 1897
218. Satnam translated by Vishav Bharti; *Jangalnama travels in a Maoist guerrilla zone*; Penguin books, 2010; p. 59

CHAPTER 25 ADDICTIONS

219. Chopra RN, Chopra GS. *The Opium smoking habit in India*, Part 1 General survey; Indian Medical Gazette, February 1938; p. 81
220. Chopra RN, Chopra GS. *Present position of The Opium smoking habit in India*, Part III General survey; Indian Medical Gazette, April 1938; p. 193
221. Chopra RN, Chopra GS. *Some country beers of India*; Indian Medical Gazette, December 1933; pp. 665-675
222. *Crombie and the Opium Question*; Indian Medical Gazette, November 1893; p. 381
223. Cullen P. *Two cases of poisoning by Majoon or Majum*; Indian Medical Gazette, June 1868; p. 131

224. Ewens GFW. *Insanity following the use of Indian Hemp*; Indian Medical Gazette; November 1904, p. 421
225. Goodall EW. *Poisoning in India*; BMJ, September 1892; p. 642
226. Homes E. *Analysis and Report Original documentary evidence concerning the use of opium in India*; BMJ, January 1894; p. 99
227. Lovell J. *The Opium War, Drugs, Dreams and the Making of China*; Picador, 2011
228. *Magic and Medicine of Plants*; Reader's Digest, 1986; pp. 12, 386
229. O'Shaughnessy WB. *On the preparations of the Indian Hemp, or Gunjah*; London, Provinces Medical Journal No. 123, January 1843; pp. 340-347
230. O'Shaughnessy WB. *On the preparations of the Indian Hemp, or Gunjah*; London, Provinces Medical Journal No. 123, February 1843; pp. 363-369.
231. *Poisoning in India*; BMJ, September 1892; p. 641
232. Basu D, Banerjee A, Thippeswamy H, Mattoo SK. *Disproportionately high rate of epileptic seizure in patients abusing dextropropoxyphene*; American Journal On Addictions, Volume 18, Number 5, August 2009, pp. 417-421.
233. Nayar PK. *Days of the Raj*; Penguin books, 2009; pp. 77, 128
234. Rangarajan LN. *Kautilya the Arthashastra*; Penguin books, 1992; pp. 66, 761.
235. Foster W. *Early travels in India 1583-1619*; Oxford university press, 1921, pp. 297-298
236. *The evidence given by Surgeon-Lieutenant Colonel Lawrie E. before the Royal Commission on Opium* on January 4th, 1894

CHAPTER 26 SEX & LONGEVITY

237. Nath R. *Private Life of the Mughals of India (1526-1803 A.D.)* Rupa & Co. 2005; pp. 128-144
238. Allbutt C. *A note on Indian Medicine*; February 1928; p. 53
239. *Mahatma Gandhi and Ayurveda* — Indian Medical Record, August 1925; Indian Medical Gazette, December 1925; pp. 592-593
240. Sutherland WD. *Charaka Samhita*- Translated into English; Published by Avinash Chandra Kaviratna, Calcutta page 186; Indian Medical Gazette, February 1919; pp. 41-50
241. Robert ES. *Ayurveda life, health and longevity*; Penguin books, 1993; p. 14.
242. Cullimore DH. *Remarks on the Therapeutic action of the Aconitum Ferox, or Indian Aconite*, BMJ, 1884; pp. 1275-1277

IN CONCLUSION

243. Satnam translated by Vishav Bharti; *Jangalnama travels in a Maoist guerrilla zone*; Penguin books, 2010; p. 59

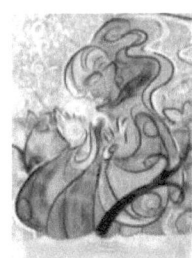

PHOTO CREDITS

1. FIG 1: Statue of the Goddess *Chamunda:* Goddess of Destruction, Epidemics, Pestilent Diseases and Famine; at a British Museum (Courtesy: Wikipedia)

2. FIG 13: Curse &Cure: Lepromatous patient sitting opposite Sun temple *Konark* (Courtesy: Ram Mohan Bajpai)

3. FIG 14: Drowning of lepromatous patient in Southern India during bathing in holy pond (Courtesy: Granger Collection, New York)

4. FIG 36: Devil's denture: Phenytoin-induced massive gum swelling in patient on long-standing therapy for epilepsy. (Courtesy: Drs Suneel Vyas, Rahul Shrivastava, YP Nagraj)

5. FIG 38: *Madak* (opium smoking pipe) – although Indians preferred to eat opium rather than to smoke it, as a culture adopted from Persia (Courtesy: Dr Inam, MD)

© Jason Green, *The Healer,* 2013

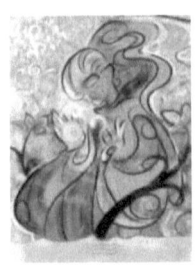

ACKNOWLEDGMENTS

This work would not have been possible without the online availability of British archival records, including *The Imperial Gazetteer of India* and British medical journals. The *Indian Medical Gazette*, preserved over the centuries in various medical libraries, have also been referred to where possible, given the constraint that these great repositories of India's medical history still await digitalization. Moreover, several authoritative monographs; scientific papers; books with extensive historical narratives of the British Raj; travelogues; and, of course, the useful nuggets of information available on *Wikipedia*, were extensively consulted during the preparation of the manuscript.

My deep gratitude to Dr. P.K. Niyogi and his family, for providing me with the Manganese poisoning enquiry committee report; to Apte, Abhimanyu, Nitin, Namrita, Pandey, Patel and Sandeep Dave, for their suggestions on the manuscript; and to Soniya, for her excellent technical support.

The support and encouragement of many friends was crucial during the writing of this book. My sincere thanks to all of them, especially to Jawwad, Pankaj, Inam, Ajim, Shakir, Rajeev, Raju, Ritu, Manu, Chinu, Chunkey, Harshit, Jagdish, Kalyan, Vishnu, Quresh, Rajesh, Abbas, Atul, Ajay and Saurabh. Last, but surely not the least, Dr (Mrs) Praneeta Sharma and Dr. Pradeep Dewangan, deserve special thanks for the many ways they have facilitated my task of writing this book.

www.ingramcontent.com/pod-product-compliance
Lightning Source LLC
Chambersburg PA
CBHW031629210526
45464CB00004B/1811